COGNITIVE-BEHAVIORAL THERAPY FOR ANXIETY DISORDERS

Guides to Individualized Evidence-Based Treatment

Jacqueline B. Persons, *Series Editor*

Providing roadmaps for managing real-world cases, volumes in this series help the clinician develop treatment plans using interventions of proven effectiveness. With an emphasis on systematic yet flexible case formulation, these hands-on guides provide powerful alternatives to one-size-fits-all approaches. Each book addresses a particular disorder or presents cutting-edge intervention strategies that can be used across a range of clinical problems.

Cognitive Therapy of Schizophrenia
David G. Kingdon and Douglas Turkington

Treating Bipolar Disorder: A Clinician's Guide to Interpersonal
and Social Rhythm Therapy
Ellen Frank

Modular Cognitive-Behavioral Therapy for Childhood Anxiety Disorders
Bruce F. Chorpita

Cognitive-Behavioral Therapy for PTSD: A Case Formulation Approach
Claudia Zayfert and Carolyn Black Becker

Cognitive-Behavioral Therapy for Adult Asperger Syndrome
Valerie L. Gaus

Cognitive-Behavioral Therapy for Anxiety Disorders: Mastering Clinical Challenges
Gillian Butler, Melanie Fennell, and Ann Hackmann

The Case Formulation Approach to Cognitive-Behavior Therapy
Jacqueline B. Persons

Mindfulness- and Acceptance-Based Behavioral Therapies in Practice
Lizabeth Roemer and Susan M. Orsillo

Cognitive-Behavioral Therapy for Anxiety Disorders
MASTERING CLINICAL CHALLENGES

Gillian Butler
Melanie Fennell
Ann Hackmann

Series Editor's Note by Jacqueline B. Persons

THE GUILFORD PRESS
New York   London

Library of Congress Cataloging-in-Publication Data

Butler, Gillian.
    Cognitive-behavioral therapy for anxiety disorders : mastering clinical
challenges / by Gillian Butler, Melanie Fennell, Ann Hackmann.
        p. ; cm.—(Guides to individualized evidence-based treatment)
    Includes bibliographical references and index.
    ISBN 978-1-59385-830-8 (hardcover : alk. paper)
        1. Anxiety disorders—Treatment. 2. Cognitive therapy. I. Fennell,
Melanie J. V. II. Hackmann, Ann. III. Title. IV. Series.
    [DNLM: 1. Anxiety Disorders—therapy. 2. Cognitive
Therapy. WM 172 B985c 2008]
    RC531.B88 2008
    616.85′ 2206—dc22

                                                             2008014217

About the Authors

Gillian Butler, PhD, a Fellow of the British Psychological Society and a Founding Fellow of the Academy of Cognitive Therapy, works for the Oxford Cognitive Therapy Centre in the United Kingdom. For 10 years she did research in Oxford helping to develop and evaluate cognitive-behavioral treatments for anxiety disorders. Dr. Butler has a special clinical interest in the use of cognitive-behavioral therapy during recovery from traumatic experiences in childhood, and runs training workshops in the United Kingdom and internationally on a wide variety of topics relevant to practitioners of cognitive-behavioral therapy. She is particularly interested in making the products of research available to the general public, and her book *Overcoming Social Anxiety and Shyness* (1999) is now available as a self-help course as well. Dr. Butler is coauthor, with Tony Hope, of *Manage Your Mind: The Mental Fitness Guide* (2nd edition; 2007) and, with Freda McManus, of *Psychology: A Very Short Introduction* (1998). She is also coeditor of the highly successful *Oxford Guide to Behavioural Experiments in Cognitive Therapy* (2004).

Melanie Fennell, PhD, is one of the pioneers of cognitive therapy in the United Kingdom. As a research therapist in Oxford University's Department of Psychiatry, she has contributed to the development of models and treatment protocols for depression and for a range of anxiety disorders. Dr. Fennell is currently a member of a team, led by Professor J. Mark G. Williams, developing mindfulness-based cognitive therapy for people suffering from recurrent depression and suicidality. A founding member of the Oxford Cognitive Therapy Centre, Dr. Fennell has written widely on cognitive-behavioral therapy for depression and low self-esteem, including the books *Overcoming Low Self-Esteem* (1999) and *Overcoming Low Self-Esteem: Self-Help Course* (2006). With colleagues from the Oxford Cognitive Therapy Centre, she was contributing author and coeditor of the *Oxford Guide to Behavioural Experiments in Cognitive Therapy* (2004). Dr. Fennell has contributed to conferences and delivered workshops in many countries. In 2002, she was voted "Most Influential Female UK Cognitive Therapist" by the membership of the British Association of Behavioural and Cognitive Psychotherapies at their 30th anniversary conference.

Ann Hackmann, PhD, is a clinical psychologist who has worked for over 20 years in a research group that specializes in the development of cognitive therapy protocols for the different anxiety disorders. She has worked as a therapist in a large number of randomized controlled trials and has done research on phenomenology of anxiety disorders and refinement of treatment strategies. Dr. Hackmann's special interest is in imagery and its relationship to memory in psychopathology, and with Emily Holmes she edited a special edition of the journal *Memory* (2004) on this topic. She was also one of the editors of the *Oxford Guide to Behavioural Experiments in Cognitive Therapy* (2004). Dr. Hackmann has also provided teaching and training in cognitive therapy in many settings in the United Kingdom and internationally, and is a Founding Fellow of the Academy of Cognitive Therapy.

Series Editor's Note

One of the mental health professional's most challenging tasks is to use findings from the research literature in a way that is thoughtful, theory guided, and responsive to the needs of the case at hand. This wonderful book by Gillian Butler, Melanie Fennell, and Ann Hackmann provides both conceptual and practical guidance to the clinician facing this task.

The evidence base underpinning treatment of the anxiety disorders has exploded in recent decades. Researchers have developed effective treatments for all of the anxiety disorders, and they are beginning to describe the psychological mechanisms underpinning the symptoms and disorders, and the process of change during effective treatment. As a result, the clinician can easily have the sense that work with individuals with anxiety disorders should proceed smoothly and quickly to a successful and long-lasting conclusion. However, this is frequently not the case. The disorder-focused protocols of the empirically supported treatments simply do not provide all the answers for all of our patients with anxiety disorders.

This book fills in many of the missing pieces. Even more important, it offers principles and illustrates a way of working that can help clinicians generate the answers they need when the protocols come up short. The authors assume that most readers are familiar with the diagnosis-specific cognitive-behavioral models and therapies. They go beyond the protocols to address common obstacles that impede work with the complex patient with an anxiety disorder. They focus particularly on difficulties that arise when avoidance, especially avoidance of affect, is extensive; when low self-esteem and comorbid depression are present; and when tolerance for uncertainty is low. The authors help clinicians accomplish thoroughgoing change that pervades cognitive, behavioral, and emotional systems. They describe how to end therapy in a way that helps patients consolidate and maintain their gains.

Although the book focuses on the complex anxiety disorders, it also provides a model of clinical work that will be useful to clinicians who work with a broad range of symptoms and problems in outpatient practice. It offers a model for using data and theory and idiographic conceptualization to guide clinical decision making. It helps the clinician work in a fully collaborative way with the patient to develop and use a formulation of the case to identify treatment targets and carry out effective interventions, and to problem-solve when initial success is not forthcoming.

These authors are truly remarkable in their ability to teach and model the integration of science, theory, and clinical experience in their clinical work. They are clearly master clinicians who are at the top of their game and are worthy models for any of us. This material is particularly useful for Americans and others outside of Great Britain because it brings us up to date with the large body of important and interesting work in the anxiety disorders in the United Kingdom that has not been disseminated as widely as its importance merits.

I am delighted to include this book in the Guides to Individualized Evidence-Based Treatment series. I am certain it will make an important contribution to the treatment of anxiety disorders in particular and to the integration of science and practice in cognitive-behavioral therapy more generally.

JACQUELINE B. PERSONS, PhD
San Francisco Bay Area Center for Cognitive Therapy

Preface

This is a book for clinicians about working with people who suffer from anxiety disorders. Cognitive-behavioral models and treatment protocols have now been developed for a range of anxiety disorders, and proved effective. This might lead clinicians to anticipate that the treatment of anxiety will be trouble free. In practice, however, even skilled and experienced clinicians experience difficulties in applying what they know, sometimes encountering problems in the application of standard methods to apparently straightforward cases. Sometimes they find that established protocols cannot satisfactorily address difficulties that arise in treating atypical or complex manifestations of anxiety. Written from a cognitive-behavioral perspective, this book addresses problems and difficulties that commonly arise during treatment and provides a wide range of practical solutions to these difficulties. We link these solutions to the theoretical foundations of cognitive therapy, and to research findings when these are relevant, and we provide illustrative examples from our experience of clinical practice. We focus on solutions that our patients have found helpful, and we attempt to explain clearly the underlying clinical principles that give them a wider applicability.

Our main aim is therefore to help clinicians to solve problems that arise in the treatment of anxiety disorders. A second but perhaps equally important goal is to help readers to draw on theoretical knowledge when seeking solutions to problems they have not previously encountered—to provide a syntax for clinical problem solving and not just a collection of unconnected techniques. In a book such as this it is impossible to address every single problem that is likely to arise during the treatment of anxiety disorders. However, it is possible to systematize solution seeking, and thus to enable practicing clinicians to use their creativity in a theoretically sound way.

STARTING POINTS: BACKGROUND KNOWLEDGE REQUIRED

We assume readers already have some experience in treating anxious people and have come across at least some of the difficulties that arise in clinical practice. Other books have focused on the basic methods and techniques of cognitive therapy for anxiety disorders, and we refer readers to the classics, such as Beck, Emery, and Greenberg (1985), and later volumes that specify further details, such as Wells (1997) and Barlow (2002).

For those seeking an introduction to the methods of cognitive therapy in general there are many excellent books available—for example, Hawton, Salkovskis, Kirk, and Clark (1989); J. S. Beck (1995); Padesky and Greenberger (1995); Simos (2002); Bennett-Levy, Butler, et al. (2004); and Westbrook, Kennerley, and Kirk (2007). Those who wish to encourage their patients to explore self-help materials about cognitive-behavioral therapy will find many useful ideas in Greenberger and Padesky (1995) and in Butler and Hope (2007). Self-help books and workbooks focusing on single disorders, which can also be used to guide therapy, include those in the excellent *Overcoming* series published by Constable & Robinson (e.g., *Overcoming Social Anxiety and Shyness* [Butler, 1999b] and *Overcoming Low Self-Esteem* [Fennell, 1999]) and in the series of workbooks on *Treatments That Work* edited by David Barlow and published by Oxford University Press (New York).

ORGANIZATION OF THIS BOOK

The book is organized into five main parts. Part I reviews current ideas and research on treating anxiety disorders. Parts II through V mirror the order in which therapy usually progresses, with each part designed to address the specific difficulties that commonly arise during that phase.

In the opening chapter, "Treating Anxiety Disorders: The State of the Art," we set the scene by summarizing current, research-based models for the specific anxiety disorders. These models provide the basis for the empirically validated treatments for these conditions, and for the specific treatment protocols that are commonly taught. Indeed, these models reflect the enormous advances that have been made in the effectiveness of anxiety treatments in the last 25 years. But this does not mean that no problems remain. Although treatment effectiveness has improved hugely, there is still some way to go. For example, until 3 or 4 years ago, at least one third of the patients in research trials for generalized anxiety disorder gained little if anything from treatment. Additionally, in most research trials a high degree of patient selection is necessary so that research findings relate to a specific, clearly defined condition and can be compared worldwide, across centers of study. In clinical practice it is not usual to apply such rigorous selection criteria, and anxious patients may come for treatment with mixed, comorbid conditions involving different types of anxiety, anxiety and depression, or anxiety in the context of one (or more) of the personality disorders. So Chapter 1 also identifies issues and questions arising about the models. It ends with a summary of the problems to which solutions will be sought in the rest of the book.

Part II (Chapters 2, 3, and 4) addresses issues related to "Deepening Understanding and Securing Engagement." Chapter 2, "Assessment: Investigating Appraisals in Depth," takes the reader immediately to the heart of the cognitive approach. Current models for the anxiety disorders focus largely (and usefully) on the specific maintaining factors for each condition (e.g., catastrophic misinterpretation of symptoms in the case of panic disorder; fear of negative evaluation by others and self-consciousness in the case of social phobia). In this chapter we discuss some of the unusual cognitive factors that may be missed in a particular patient, and which may therefore interfere with progress. Theory tells us that understanding cognitive factors in depth is essential to identifying appropriate treatment targets. Methods for doing so are described in detail here.

Chapter 3, "Case Formulation: Making Sense of Complexity," acknowledges the difficulty of constructing clear, theoretically sound formulations when faced with atypical or complex cases. The principles for work on formulation are clarified, placing a considerable degree of emphasis on parsimony. Atypical and complex cases are difficult to formulate, and there is a risk that, when faced with a difficulty, therapists also construct increasingly complex case formulations. The end product may then become difficult to understand, and difficult for the patient and the therapist to use as a basis for decisions about how to intervene. It is argued here, consistent with the argument in Chapter 2 on assessment, that it is particularly important to learn to think about deeper levels of patient cognition—about beliefs as well as about thoughts and assumptions. Strategies to help clinicians do this, and to use this information in their formulation work, are described and illustrated.

Once assessment and formulation are in place, cognitive-behavioral change methods can be introduced. However, to engage effectively in this work, patients need to be able to stand back far enough from old patterns of thought to recognize them (even if only in theory) as learned opinions, rather than as fact. Chapter 4, "Decentering from Thoughts: Achieving Objectivity," addresses the problem of subjectivity, when patients experience their habitual thought patterns as reflections of objective truth and so are unable or unwilling to engage in the process of change.

Part III (Chapters 5 and 6) focuses on "Facilitating Emotional Processing." Even when assessment, formulation, and engagement in therapy are successfully in place, and work with cognitive-behavioral strategies has begun, difficulties can arise in ensuring that transformation occurs on all levels—cognitive, behavioral, and emotional. Desynchronous change (change that occurs at one level but not simultaneously at other levels) is likely to be transitory (e.g., Rachman, 1980), and therapists need to include in their clinical repertoires methods other than the verbal process of guided discovery that we recognize as being at the heart of cognitive therapy. Chapter 5, "Bringing About Lasting Change at the Deepest Level," reflects on common processes underlying different cognitive techniques and on theoretical models of emotional processing. It recognizes that meanings may be hard to identify, to express, and to represent in words, and that they may be encapsulated in memories, or in symbolic representations such as images and metaphors. Here strategies for working with images, memory, and metaphor are carefully described so that readers can discover how to use them effectively when working on meanings that are otherwise resistant to change. Pursuing the same theme, Chapter 6, "The Role of Behavioral Experiments," outlines the principles underlying the creation of successful behavioral experiments. It explains in detail how to use this powerful experiential method, in which changes in behavior are closely linked to changes in cognition and affect, to achieve lasting whole-person change.

Part IV, "Overcoming Three Major Obstacles to Progress" (Chapters 7, 8, and 9), deals with three major obstacles that commonly interfere with progress: emotional avoidance, enduring negative perspectives on the self, and intolerance of uncertainty. In Chapter 7, "Avoidance of Affect," we focus on the difficulties some patients have in expressing, and even in experiencing, feelings of anxiety. Chapter 8, "Low Self-Esteem," focuses on cases where anxiety forms part of a more complex picture, where comorbid anxiety and depression have their roots in long-standing low self-esteem. The chapter suggests that these linked problems can be parsimoniously addressed by using a cognitive model of low self-esteem that incorporates all three. In Chapter 9, "Dealing with Uncertainty," we consider more general attitudes that can determine responses to anxiety and to the problems that anxiety brings. We also pay attention here to some of the uncertainties that remain for us as clinicians, despite all the advances that have been made in our ability to help people who suffer from anxiety.

Part V (Chapter 10) closes the book with "Ending Treatment Productively." This offers a systematic approach to termination to help ensure that the new learning gained in therapy is not lost once treatment ends. Chapter 10, "Creating a Therapy 'Blueprint,' " is constructed to help readers to prepare themselves as well as their patients for a future that will be full of uncertainties.

THEMES RUNNING THROUGH THE BOOK

In practice, the separation of methods and topics into discrete categories, though necessary for the purposes of clarity, is also artificial. We are well aware, for example, that behavioral experiments can be used to help create formulations, that images may be usefully explored during the assessment phase, and so on. Nevertheless, we have chosen the particular topics of our chapters with care, drawing on our own clinical knowledge of the problems that commonly interfere with smooth progress when we treat anxiety. We have arranged the chapters to reflect the usual order of treatment, in order to help readers to find ideas that will help them when they are faced with particular dilemmas. Each chapter can be used on its own, as a resource. Within each chapter a range of ideas is provided to help refine methods of therapy, and to explain how to use them to best advantage in difficult circumstances.

Reading the book as a whole, however, will reveal five recurring themes. First is the style of cognitive therapy. We emphasize repeatedly the value of explicitness, collaboration, the Socratic method, and the openness of mind that is necessary when we explore, question, and test cognitions. We believe that this style in itself carries therapeutic weight. Second, as therapists and as researchers, we have always been aware of the importance of the therapeutic relationship and the need to pay close attention to the processes that occur during a complex course of therapy. There are many other books on the therapeutic relationship, so we have not devoted a specific chapter to it here but rather have illustrated our attitudes and behavior through numerous clinical illustrations. Our third theme is the importance of thinking about meaning—about the many ways in which it can be represented; about beliefs as well as about surface-level cognitions. This theme recurs constantly as we pursue our clinical work, and in our discussions of issues and problems, with each other and with other colleagues. Personal meanings can be highly idiosyncratic, and not always easily represented in the established models that provided our starting point. We believe that an elaborated understanding of the complexity of meaning is central to the theory that underpins cognitive therapy and provides a rich source of ideas about how to proceed when standard methods appear to fail. The fourth theme reflects the need to aim, during therapy, for full emotional processing—for "whole-system" change. The fifth and final theme is more specific to working with anxiety disorders. The suggestions for dealing with difficulties in clinical practice are held together by three general principles: to encourage curiosity rather than control; to increase flexibility (and reduce rigidity); and to help people to face, accept, and explore when they feel anxious, rather than seeking protection through avoidance or safety behaviors. Developing, modeling, and helping patients to adopt an accepting attitude toward uncertainty provides a constructive and confidence-building context within which to apply these ideas.

ABOUT THE AUTHORS

The three authors of this book bring together a unique combination of ideas. All three of us received a broad clinical training, with a clear behavioral component, before the "cognitive revolution" began. Then, having trained as cognitive therapists early in the 1980s, we all spent many years working in a research capacity at the University of Oxford, acting as therapists in randomized controlled trials and contributing to the development and evaluation of specific applications of cognitive-behavioral therapy. Gillian Butler's research originally focused on developing cognitive methods for the treatment of social phobia and generalized anxiety disorder, and on exploring the cognitive processes linked to anxiety. Subsequently, she has focused clinically on working with complex, and apparently treatment-resistant, problems such as those that follow a history of neglect or abuse during childhood. She has special interests in the relationship between theory and practice, for example, in case formulation work, and also in the development of cognitive methods for working with people who have problems of identity. Melanie Fennell started her research career in Oxford by focusing on cognitive therapy for depression, developed a ground-breaking approach to problems of self-esteem, and her current research focuses on evaluating the use of mindfulness-based cognitive therapy. On the way, she also contributed to research on generalized anxiety disorder, social phobia, and posttraumatic stress disorder (PTSD). Ann Hackmann has worked in the Anxiety Disorders Research Group at Oxford and at the Institute of Psychiatry in London, contributing to research on a number of anxiety disorders, including panic disorder, agoraphobia, health anxiety, social phobia, and PTSD. Throughout, she has maintained a special interest in the patients' experience of imagery, and her current research continues to explore issues concerning the pervasiveness of imagery, its links to memory, and the uses therapists can make of it. All three authors are also experienced supervisors and trainers of cognitive-behavioral therapy, and continue to run advanced workshops on new developments in cognitive therapy. This combination of theoretical knowledge, clinical experience, and research expertise focuses here on finding theoretically based and practical solutions to problems that arise during the treatment of anxiety disorders.

Contents

PART I
SETTING THE SCENE

ONE

Treating Anxiety Disorders
The State of the Art

This is a very exciting moment in the development of cognitive therapy for the anxiety disorders. Initially the cognitive-behavioral perspective on anxiety was relatively generic. Then specific models proliferated, bringing increased diversity and specificity. Now a new synthesis is emerging, with increasing appreciation of common transdiagnostic processes, targets, and procedures.

Each of these perspectives throws light on the problem of anxiety, and each has proved helpful in the evolution of treatment strategies. This book aims to explore further the synthesis that is currently emerging and extend the range of the diagnosis-based models and protocols. We do this by explicitly exploring the areas that, by design, disorder-specific models do not address such as comorbidity, avoidance of affect, low self-esteem, and other factors.

COGNITIVE THERAPY AND ANXIETY

Shortly after completing their book on cognitive therapy of depression (Beck, Rush, Shaw, & Emery, 1979), Beck and his colleagues (1985) developed a treatment manual for anxiety. A basic tenet was that the thinking present in anxiety could be differentiated from that present in depression: the "cognitive specificity" hypothesis. Depression was seen to be concerned with loss, whereas anxiety involved the perception of physical or psychosocial threat, together with an underestimate of coping and rescue factors. Common features of anxiety disorders were described, and there was some differentiation of the particular thematic content and maintenance processes within specific disorders. However, the main thrust was to develop a relatively transdiagnostic approach to anxiety, and an understanding of processes and themes common to different anxiety disorders. Afterwards, how these commonalities were manifested in each of the anxiety disorders specified in the *Diagnostic and Statistical Manual of Mental Disorders* (DSM) could be worked out in detail.

This careful work, closely tied to direct clinical observation, provided the context for the development of specific cognitive models for the anxiety disorders. One of the earliest was Clark's (1986) cognitive model of panic. Over a period of 20 years, there has been increasing precision and refinement in our understanding of the specific content of the thinking in different disorders, the links between various features of the anxiety disorders, and the exact nature of the vicious circles that maintain them. This sharpening of focus has allowed us to formulate and treat anxiety disorders with more accuracy, efficacy, and sophistication. Central mechanisms and associated treatment objectives have been proposed for each disorder, and the refinement of our knowledge of these targets and of effective procedures for tackling them continues (Clark, 1999, 2004).

Most familiar to us are the models and treatment protocols initially developed in Oxford, England, in the development and evaluation of which we were closely involved. These naturally provide the starting place for many of the arguments presented in this book, although we also draw on a wealth of ideas presented by others, including research groups led by Borkovec, Foa, Heimberg, Barlow, Freeston, Ost, Rachman, Rapee, Arntz, Wells, and van der Hout. In addition, a growing body of research has confirmed the clinical utility of disorder-specific models and treatments, while experimental investigations of hypothesized underlying processes have illuminated the development and maintenance of anxiety. A solid evidence base has accumulated, including randomized controlled outcome trials (RCTs) of treatments derived from the models in many of the disorders. As a consequence, as Clark (2004) notes, observed effect sizes in treatment trials have increased substantially in the last 20 years.

In research trials treatment derived from specific models for cases with one main anxiety disorder is typically efficient and highly effective, with good results at follow-up. The treatment usually requires not more than 20 hours with the therapist, with shorter packages also having been shown to produce very good results in 5 hours or fewer in some cases (e.g., panic disorders; Clark et al., 1999).

Increasing clarity concerning particular cognitive and behavioral features specific to each disorder has led to increased clarity about treatment targets and procedures, and hence to specific protocols such as those described by Wells (1997) and Simos (2002). It has also given rise to a greater understanding of underlying processes. For example, Salkovskis (1991, 1996) hypothesized that anxious patients fail to update old perspectives because, even if they expose themselves to feared situations, they take unnecessary precautions (safety-seeking behaviors, often called "safety behaviors") to prevent bad things from happening, and so never have the opportunity to discover that their expectations are inaccurate. With this understanding, the therapist is able to encourage patients to test predictions by dropping safety behaviors and observing and reflecting on the results. Thus behavioral experiments pave the way for enhancement of belief change and associated shifts in affect, compared to the possibly more gradual results of repeated situational exposure (Bennett-Levy, Butler, et al., 2004; Salkovskis, Clark, Hackmann, Wells, & Gelder, 1999; Salkovskis, Hackmann, Wells, Gelder, & Clark, 2007).

Such developments led to the elaboration of the models of disorders. For example, Clark's (1986) original model of panic now incorporates several further maintenance cycles, and thus extra targets for treatment, that is, avoidance, safety-seeking behaviors, and selective attention to internal cues (Clark, 1988; Salkovskis, 1991; Wells, 1997).

Thus, the elaboration of cognitive models of the anxiety disorders can be seen as a work in progress, where further refinement is possible, as in the case of the recently established Obsessive–Compulsive Cognitions Working Group (OCCWG; 1997).

The real-world clinical relevance of RCTs carried out in centers of excellence (often university based) has been hotly debated. Critics often suggest that the constraints of working in a research setting imply that the results of clinical trials cannot usefully be generalized to patients seen in ordinary mental health care facilities. However, this view may underestimate the severity of problems encountered in many RCTs, and the degree of creative flexibility required of therapists if they are to tailor models and treatment protocols to the endless, rich variety of real patients' lives and experiences.

It is true that, in research trials, a relatively homogeneous group of patients is deliberately selected to diminish extraneous sources of variance, and to ensure a good "fit" between patient and therapy (perhaps particularly important with innovative and still relatively untested approaches). Nevertheless, each patient presents a different picture, and idiographic formulation (using the model under investigation as a foundation) has always guided the work of research cognitive therapists. Results from efficacy trials of this nature can then become a basis for investigations that set out to explore the effectiveness of treatments initially tested with relatively homogeneous groups in a broader, less tightly selected patient population (e.g., Westbrook & Kirk, 2005).

In ordinary clinical practice therapists often cannot select their patients. Nonetheless, they can fruitfully draw on the careful detail and precision of diagnosis-specific models. However, therapists in mental health care services are also constrained by lack of resources and often encounter caseloads of clinical complexity, severity, and high comorbidity (including personality disorder). This means that therapists are still faced by difficulties and dilemmas that existing specific models and protocols are not designed to address, and thus may not entirely resolve. This book attempts to address some of these difficulties and dilemmas.

A TRANSDIAGNOSTIC VIEW OF UNDERLYING COGNITIVE AND BEHAVIORAL PROCESSES

As disorder-specific models and protocols for anxiety were developed and tested, an observation emerged that anxiety disorders, whatever the precise focus of their central concerns, shared common underlying processes, and thus (at least to some degree) commonalities in effective treatment interventions. These common interventions included dropping safety-seeking behaviors, decreasing avoidance, carrying out behavioral experiments, redirecting attention, challenging negative cognitions, cutting out rumination and worry, and reflecting on input from memory in the form of images and memories. Thus our increasing understanding of separate anxiety disorders may be leading toward a new and more sophisticated synthesis.

This perspective was examined by Harvey, Watkins, Mansell, and Shafran (2004), who synthesized emerging evidence for commonalities in underlying processes across many types of disorder (i.e., not just in the anxiety disorders). Harvey et al. examined the following cognitive and behavioral processes in a number of specific disorders, and summarized and evaluated experimental evidence for their influence on affective disturbance:

- Selective *attention*, which can be controlled or automatic, and directed toward concern-related internal or external stimuli, including sources of safety.
- Explicit and implicit selective *memory*, recurrent memory, overgeneral memory, avoidant encoding and retrieval, working memory, and memory distrust.
- A wide range of *reasoning* processes, including interpretation, expectancy, attributional and emotional reasoning. Many of these reasoning processes map onto the classic "cognitive distortions" or logical errors described in cognitive therapy, such as personalization, all-or-nothing thinking, mind reading, fortune telling, and so on.
- Recurrent *thinking* (i.e., rumination and worry), and associated positive and negative meta-cognitive beliefs (beliefs about worry and other mental events and processes).
- Avoidance and safety-seeking *behaviors*, designed to avert danger and reduce threat, but unfortunately feeding into preoccupation, and leaving negative beliefs untested.

Evidence has suggested that some (but not all) of these processes are ubiquitous in the anxiety disorders. Indeed, they are repeatedly referred to in the information concerning the specific anxiety disorders that follows this section.

Harvey and colleagues (2004) considered treatment implications, and described possible procedures for targeting different processes across disorders. A similar thrust is evident in the work of Mogg and Bradley (2004) on a cognitive-motivational analysis of anxiety, where commonalities across disorders were examined. In addition, a cross-diagnostic comparison was made concerning imagery and its relationship to memory in articles in a recent special issue of *Memory* (Conway, Meares, & Standart, 2004; Hackmann & Holmes, 2004).

Given the human tendency toward dichotomous thinking (there are two ways of seeing this—my way, and the wrong way), a danger arises here: a tension between differentiation and specificity on one hand, and synthesis and commonality on the other. It would be to our detriment as clinicians to reject disorder-specific models and treatment protocols as narrow, rigid, and irrelevant to the real world of clinical practice. Their authors have teased out the essence of different anxiety disorders and prompt us carefully to analyze the nature of the anxieties our patients confront, tracking unhelpful sequences and illuminating connections. With their help, we can more readily target our treatment interventions with precision. This is why we use them as our starting point in this book. Equally, however, it would be to our detriment to ignore common processes across anxiety disorders because they can help us and our patients to understand how one problem relates to another, and to broader background issues (schemas, beliefs). Thus learning in one area can productively generalize to others, with corresponding gains in the depth and breadth of change. Discerning inclusiveness may thus benefit us more than rejection of either possibility: both/and may be more helpful to our patients than either/or.

Thus, our book starts from the assumption that current specific theoretical models and protocols for the anxiety disorders provide extremely useful templates for treatment and should inform and guide our real-world clinical practice in treating anxiety disorders when relevant. Our aim is not to replace them but rather to explain how we can supplement or enhance their application and widen understanding (without sacrificing sharpness of focus) in cases where a single model might fall short.

In the descriptions below we emphasize strategies with a rationale that involves changing meanings in direct or more indirect ways, as the central thesis of cognitive therapy is that meaning is the engine that drives our reactions.

CURRENT MODELS AND PROTOCOLS

Here we present a brief synthesis of current models and protocols on which we draw for work in each of the anxiety disorders. Each section begins with a definition of the disorder, based on DSM-IV-TR (American Psychiatric Association [APA], 2000). Then we present a cognitive understanding of the essence of the disorder, followed by a description of key treatment strategies, before moving on to potential complicating factors. Fuller descriptions of potential protocols and specific treatment strategies for each anxiety disorder can be found in Hawton, Salkovskis, Kirk, and Clark (1989); Simos (2002); Wells (1997); Bennett-Levy, Butler, and colleagues (2004); Barlow (1988); and Leahy and Hollon (2000). The material we draw on can also be examined in more depth by consulting the references in Table 1.1.

Panic Disorder and Agoraphobia

A panic attack is a sudden increase in anxiety accompanied by four or more of a list of symptoms, mostly of autonomic arousal. The term "panic disorder" is reserved for a condition in which individuals have recurrent panic attacks, some of which are unexpected.

Agoraphobia is defined as anxiety about being in situations in which escape would be embarrassing, or help unavailable in the case of a panic attack, or panic-like symptoms. It is always defined in relation to panic disorder. Most patients with panic disorder have some degree of agoraphobic avoidance.

TABLE 1.1. References Relating to Models and Protocols for the Anxiety Disorders

Anxiety disorder	References
Panic disorder and agoraphobia	Clark (1986, 1988); Hackmann (1998a); Salkovskis (1991); Wells (1997)
Health anxiety	Salkovskis & Warwick (1986); Warwick & Salkovskis (1990); Wells & Hackmann (1993)
Social phobia	Clark (2004); Clark & Wells (1995); Wells & Clark (1997)
Obsessive–compulsive disorder	Freeston, Rheaume, & Ladouceur (1996); Salkovskis (1985); Salkovskis, Forrester, et al. (1999); Wells (1997)
Generalized anxiety disorder	Borkovec & Newman (1998); Ladouceur et al. (2000); Newman & Borkovec (2002); Wells (1997, 2000, 2002)
Specific phobia	Kirk & Rouf (2004)
Posttraumatic stress disorder	Brewin (2001); Ehlers & Clark (2000)

A Cognitive Understanding of Panic Disorder and Agoraphobia

The best-known cognitive model is that of Clark (1986). The model proposes that people who suffer from recurrent (unexpected) panic attacks have a relatively enduring tendency to misinterpret bodily sensations as indicating *imminent* physical or mental catastrophe such as fainting, going crazy, having a heart attack, suffocating, dying, or being suddenly incapacitated in some other way. The sensations that are misinterpreted are mainly signs of autonomic arousal. The catastrophic misinterpretations generate anxiety, the symptoms of which trigger fresh catastrophic thoughts, followed by increased anxiety. In later papers on panic disorder Salkovskis emphasized the role played by safety-seeking behaviors (unnecessary precautions) in maintaining such catastrophic interpretations (e.g., Salkovskis, Clark, et al., 1999).

There can be some overlap with health anxiety or hypochondriasis, in which the feared catastrophe is seen as likely to occur at some time in the future, when the current symptoms of hypothesized disease ultimately culminate in severe illness or death.

We know of no explicit attempts to elaborate the cognitive model further, to take into account apparent differences in the presentation of patients with more severe agoraphobic avoidance, although a review of the literature suggests this might need to incorporate interpersonal beliefs concerning perceived coping and rescue factors (Chambless & Goldstein, 1982; Hackmann, 1998a; Salkovskis & Hackmann, 1997). This is discussed below, under common complicating factors.

Key Maintaining Processes

- Catastrophic misinterpretations of bodily sensations (mainly those of autonomic arousal).
- Biased attention to concern-related bodily sensations (e.g., heart rate or breathlessness).
- Safety behaviors, with a meaningful relationship to concerns (Salkovskis, Clark, & Gelder, 1996). For example, someone who experiences a pounding heart may fear a heart attack and sit or lie down, whereas someone who is afraid of becoming paralyzed with fear might try to keep moving.
- Avoidance of potential panic triggers, especially in people with agoraphobia.

Treatment Strategies

- Analysis of recent, specific instances of panic, and the construction of the vicious circle model, using the patient's own material. Links are made between symptoms and feared catastrophes, and between catastrophic thoughts, understandable increases in anxiety, and safety-seeking behaviors.
- The patient collaborates with the therapist in reaching a shared understanding of the true (harmless) causes of the feared symptoms. Benign explanations are generated via guided discovery and provision of new information. Behavioral experiments are used to validate these new ideas (e.g., the patient demonstrates how he or she breathes deeply when trying to stay calm and discovers that deep breaths make the dizziness worse).

- The patient is encouraged to do behavioral experiments to test the possible (actually benign) consequences if symptoms are not controlled (e.g., the patient dresses very warmly and stays in a very hot room for a stretch of time, to discover that being hot does not lead to fainting).
- At a later stage attempts are made to discover triggers for unexpected attacks, even if they are hard to spot. An example might be the patient realizing that an episode of rapid heartbeats might have been triggered by three cups of coffee, rather than heart disease. This helps consolidate an alternative, benign perspective on symptoms of panic.

In some approaches exposure to interoceptive and extraceptive stimuli is encouraged, with an exposure and habituation rationale, after some cognitive restructuring (e.g., Barlow, 1988; Barlow, Craske, Cerny, & Klosko, 1989). In Clark's (1986) approach cognitive restructuring and exposure are more closely integrated, using a sequence of behavioral experiments within and outside the therapy office (see Chapter 6). The rationale here is derived from Kolb's (1984) learning circle. These two methods of delivering exposure after some cognitive restructuring have not been compared directly, except in an experimental investigation (Salkovskis, Clark, et al., 1999) and a small treatment trial for agoraphobia (Salkovskis et al., 2007). In both cases framing the exposure as a set of behavioral experiments produced a more rapid decline in anxiety than an equivalent amount of *in-vivo* exposure with a habituation rationale.

Treatment of panic disorder has been shown to be very successful in patients with mild to moderate agoraphobic avoidance (Clark et al., 1994, 1999). This treatment is described more fully in Wells (1997), Simos (2002), and Bennett-Levy, Butler, and colleagues (2004).

Common Complicating Factors

In more severe cases (particularly if there is extensive agoraphobic avoidance) there is often comorbidity, including severe depression and substance abuse, and avoidant and dependent personality traits may be evident. The literature suggests concurrent separation anxiety, impaired assertiveness, social evaluative concerns, and low levels of perceived self-sufficiency and self-efficacy may be more common in patients with more severe agoraphobia. For detailed reviews, see Salkovskis and Hackmann (1997) and Hackmann (1998a). Careful assessment and formulation are necessary (Chapters 2 and 3), and engagement is crucial (Chapter 4).

In addition to having an enduring tendency to misinterpret bodily sensations as indicating an imminent catastrophe, patients may be concerned that should this occur they would be unable to cope with the interpersonal consequences of being taken ill in certain places, and would not find others willing to rescue or protect them (Hoffart, Hackmann, & Sexton, 2006). Such themes have been found in the images of those suffering from agoraphobia, and these frequently echo the content of traumatic early memories reported by the same patients, of childhood separations, abuse, neglect, and/or lack of protection (Day, Holmes, & Hackmann, 2004). It may be advisable to work on these early memories if they encapsulate current core beliefs (Chapter 5). Social evaluative concerns are often prominent, so aspects of the treatment of social phobia may be utilized.

The panic disorder model can be extended where relevant to incorporate the interpersonal dimensions of the problem. A wide range of beliefs about the self, other people, and the world may be maintaining situational avoidance. This avoidance may be maintained by automatically triggered memories of panic attacks that occurred in similar situations, as well as images with input from traumatic experiences. Behavioral experiments with the therapist can help the patient to distinguish between the past and the present and check out how other people would really react if they had a panic attack (Chapters 5 and 6).

Cognitive and emotional avoidance may also play a part. It may be difficult to identify symptoms and catastrophic misinterpretations where there is marked avoidance of affect and feared situations (see Chapter 7). It may be necessary to target depression and low self-esteem (Chapter 8). Thus the treatment of panic disorder with moderate or severe agoraphobia may require a broader focus than treatment of panic disorder without significant agoraphobic avoidance.

Health Anxiety

"Health anxiety" (or hypochondriasis) is defined as a preoccupation with the fear of having, or a belief that one has a serious disease, and a preoccupation with bodily symptoms. Other criteria are that the problem persists despite medical reassurance, causes significant distress or impaired functioning, and has lasted for at least 6 months. Hypochondriasis is classified as a somatoform disorder rather than an anxiety disorder in DSM-IV-TR. However, because this disorder involves anxiety about health, it makes sense to incorporate observations on health anxiety here. Health anxiety causes a great deal of distress to patients and to those trying to help them. Patients believe that they have serious health problems that are not receiving appropriate diagnosis or treatment, leading to repeated consultations and strained relationships with medical practitioners, and frequent requests for reassurance from helpers.

A Cognitive Understanding of Health Anxiety

Salkovskis and Warwick (1986) and Warwick and Salkovskis (1990) devised a specific model for health anxiety, which reflects how people perceive their bodily changes as more dangerous than they actually are. Health-anxious patients fear physical or mental catastrophe in a similar way to patients with panic disorder. A key difference is the time frame, with health-anxious patients fearing catastrophe in the future, and those with panic disorder fearing immediate catastrophe. As might be expected, there is significant comorbidity between panic disorder and hypochondriasis.

Assumptions about illness, symptoms, and health behaviors (such as checking for symptoms or frequent medical consultations) often have roots in past experience. This includes illness and medical treatment of self, friends, and family. Sensational media coverage of medical mismanagement may reinforce the person's assumptions and sense of vulnerability (Silver, Sanders, Morrison, & Cowey, 2004).

Key cognitions in health anxiety include beliefs about symptoms and sensations indicating disease, and the need to be vigilant; beliefs about the importance of tests to establish diagnosis; beliefs about the importance of checking and reassurance; and beliefs about the effects of stress on health (resulting in an overlap with panic disorder).

Key Maintaining Processes

- Checking and scanning the body for possible signs and symptoms.
- Symptom focusing can lead directly to bodily changes: for example, repeated checking for lumps may lead to soreness, providing fresh evidence of illness. The perception of threat leads to an increase in autonomic arousal that can be interpreted as signs of a disease.
- Repeated reassurance seeking, including frequent medical consultations and requests for tests. This may lead to unnecessary tests and interventions, and ambiguous information from medical sources.
- Exaggerated beliefs, arbitrary inference, and selective attention can result in a confirmatory bias and lead people to selectively notice and remember information consistent with their negative beliefs that would normally be ignored.
- Avoidance (in some cases) of doctors, medical information on TV or in books, and so on.

Treatment Strategies

- Engagement involves helping the patient to agree to testing Theory 2 ("This is an anxiety problem") rather than Theory 1 ("I have a serious health problem"), for a sustained period (see Chapter 4, p. 76, for a fuller exposition of this important preparation for treatment).
- A model of potential maintenance processes in health anxiety is drawn out, using the patient's own material.
- A series of behavioral experiments are carried out to test the short- and long-term effects of checking, scanning, reassurance seeking, medical consultations, and avoidance. These experiments usually generate the realization that these safety behaviors are maintaining rather than reducing anxiety. This new understanding can be conveyed to carers, who may have inadvertently colluded with unhelpful behavior.
- Patients may have beliefs about the deleterious effects of worrying (or not worrying) about health, and about the need for repeated medical tests. New information can be provided and augmented by behavioral experiments including surveys to discover the opinions of others on such matters. Full details of a range of possible experiments are given in Bennett-Levy, Butler, and colleagues (2004) and Wells (1997).

Common Complicating Factors

The significant overlap with panic disorder may mean that panic should be separately addressed. This is often a good place to start because it helps to build an alternative, anxiety-based model to set against the belief that the problem is real physical danger. In addition, the immediate threat of catastrophe makes predictions easier to test than those in hypochondriasis, where the imagined catastrophe may lie in the far future. Making progress in understanding and overcoming panic attacks instills hope and strengthens an alternative, benign perspective.

Wells and Hackmann (1993) described the content of images and associated beliefs in people with health anxiety, which incorporates exaggerated perceptions of the likely cost of illness, and underestimation of coping and rescue factors. Some examples are that illness could lead to abandonment by others, or that death could lead to hell, or eternal loneliness. Thus, as in the study on agoraphobia reported above, it appears that individuals with health anxiety may fear not only illness and death, but also the wider implications of these events. This is in accord with the observation that people with health anxiety are often lacking in self-esteem and may have interpersonal problems (Silver et al., 2004). Work on health anxiety may need to focus on factors such as low self-esteem (see Chapter 8).

In addition, Wells and Hackmann (1993) noted that the images often appeared to reflect the content of earlier adverse memories, which carried negative, personal meanings. It has been observed that assumptions about illness and death have sometimes arisen because of traumatic past illness experiences. This suggests that interventions targeting intrusive memories may be beneficial (see Chapter 5). In addition, other work may need to be done around assumptions and core beliefs underlying low self-esteem (see Chapter 8). For example, patients who believe they are unlovable may feel that no one will look after them if they become ill, making this a fearful prospect.

Silver and colleagues (2004) and Wells and Hackmann (1993) described superstitious thinking (including thought–action fusion) in health anxiety, manifest in beliefs such as "If I think about illness I will get ill," "If I picture myself looking well I will tempt fate," or "If I imagine myself dead I will die." Other metacognitive beliefs are also apparent—for example, "If I don't control my thoughts I might go mad," "Worrying about cancer makes it more likely I will get it," "If I don't worry about my health, something will go wrong," or "Worrying will help me be prepared if I become ill." In this way, health-anxious patients are similar to patients who have generalized anxiety disorder (GAD) or obsessive–compulsive disorder (OCD), and similar tactics for working with their positive and negative metacognitive beliefs may be useful (Wells, 1997).

Finally, people with health anxiety may engage in avoidance of affect, and this may need attention in its own right (see Chapter 7).

Social Phobia

In DSM-IV-TR social phobia is defined as a marked or persistent fear of one or more social or performance situations in which the person is exposed to unfamiliar people, and to possible scrutiny. The person fears that he or she will show anxiety symptoms, or act in a way that will be embarrassing or humiliating.

A Cognitive Understanding of Social Phobia

A cognitive model of social phobia was advanced by Clark and Wells (1995) and subsequently elaborated by Wells and Clark (1997). Another model was described by Rapee and Heimberg (1997). It is suggested that people with social phobia perceive danger in social situations, leading them to engage in self-processing and avoidance. This increases self-consciousness and anxiety, interferes with performance, and maintains a negative impression of the self.

People with social phobia fear rejection or humiliation, in social situations, and there is a theme of concern about acceptability. They have a distorted impression of how they come across to others. Some have an unstable sense of self: They may feel quite good about themselves when alone or in the company of those they trust, but their confidence evaporates in the face of strangers. Others suffer from more pervasive low self-esteem. There are also variations in beliefs about others, and the extent to which they are perceived as intrinsically uncaring or hostile.

Key Maintaining Processes

- Selective attention to the self (self-processing) appears to play an important role in social phobia. Under threat of rejection, people focus on their own anxiety symptoms and behavior, attending to mental images that are negative and distorted (Hackmann, Surawy, & Clark, 1998).
- Safety behaviors (designed to help one present the self more favorably) have the effect of enhancing self-focus, and interfering with performance. Examples are trying to control shaking by tensing up while holding a cup or pen, or planning every utterance in advance while trying to follow a conversation.
- Extensive (biased) anticipatory and postevent processing involves a review of past and possible future failures in social situations, and further lowering of confidence.
- Avoidance is also usually quite extensive and again prevents disconfirmation of beliefs.

Treatment Strategies

- A cognitive model indicating possible maintenance processes is drawn up, using the patient's own observations of recent, specific examples of the problem.
- During treatment, the deleterious effects of safety behaviors and self-processing are examined. Behavioral experiments are carried out in which patients are first invited to try talking to someone with and without safety behaviors and focus on the self and are videotaped while doing this. They then compare how they think they came across with how they really looked, using self-ratings, video feedback, and feedback from others. This challenges the distorted image or impression of the self and ushers in a more kindly perspective. They also usually observe that they feel less anxious and come across better when dropping their safety behaviors.
- Further behavioral experiments including surveys of the opinions of others concerning blushing, shaking, and so on provide opportunities to operationalize and test beliefs about the likely reactions of others, should the persons with social phobia drop their safety behaviors and avoidance.
- Finally more experiments may be conducted during which patients "broaden the bandwidth" by testing what happens if they actually exaggerate the very symptoms they have been trying to hide. This can be modeled first by the therapist.
- Having challenged their assumptions, patients may also need to use some schema-focused therapy techniques (e.g., positive data logs) to challenge their core beliefs.

Comprehensive descriptions of how to carefully set up a useful sequence of behavioral experiments in the treatment of social phobia are provided by Butler and Hackmann (2004), Butler (1999b), and Wells (1997).

Common Complicating Factors

Social phobia is often comorbid with GAD, substance abuse, and/or avoidant personality traits. As in the other anxiety disorders, depression is common. Low self-esteem and hopelessness can lead to a rapid dissipation of the results of positive findings from behavioral experiments. They may also undermine the person's motivation to undertake homework assignments and record the results. Studies suggest that many people with social phobias have suffered rejection, bullying, and excessive criticism in the past, and also that their current images of themselves in social situations have much in common with upsetting memories of these events (Hackmann, Clark, & McManus, 2000). People with social phobia may also be lacking in a repertoire of appropriate responses to rejection, with which they might defend themselves and their self-esteem. Such observations suggest that depression and hopelessness may also need to be tackled. Again, work on self-esteem (see Chapter 8) may also enhance results of treatment. Padesky's "assertive defense of the self" can be an empowering adjunct to treatment (Padesky, 1997, and see Chapter 8, pp. 169, 173). In addition, interventions aimed at challenging the meaning of distressing memories of bullying, rejection, and past criticism may be beneficial (see Chapter 5; and also Wild, Hackmann, & Clark, 2007). Compassionate mind training may also be beneficial where the patient is very self-critical (Gilbert, 2005a).

It may take time to build trust so that people can be clear and specific about how they see themselves, how other people might react, and the content of distressing early memories. Initially patients may avoid thinking or talking about such material because of associated shame. However, without this specificity, treatment will lack focus (see Chapters 2 and 7).

Specific Phobias

A specific phobia is defined as a persistent fear of an object or situation, exposure to which leads to immediate anxiety or even panic. Levels of fear are related to proximity, and to appraisals of ability to escape. Sufferers appreciate that the level of fear is unreasonable but feel compelled to avoid the phobic situation, or else endure it with excessive anxiety. Phobic situations or objects may be categorized as one of five subtypes: animals, natural environment (e.g., thunder), blood/injury, situational (e.g., elevators), or atypical.

A Cognitive Understanding of Specific Phobias

Phobic anxiety has been construed as a rational response in a situation misperceived as dangerous because of biases in interpretation, perception, and memory. It has been proposed that careful identification of cognitions allows for precisely targeted interventions (Kirk & Rouf, 2004).

These cognitions may include overestimates of the probability of harm in the phobic situation, underestimates of personal ability to cope, and of potential rescue factors. In addition, there may be negative self-judgments about what it means to have the phobia, and what others will think about it. People may feel that they will never overcome their phobias, which can lead to hopelessness and loss of self-esteem.

Exposure has been considered an effective procedure in the treatment of phobias for many years. In many cases a single, long session of exposure treatment can deliver good results (Ost, 1997). However, it has been argued that exposure is only effective if cognitive change occurs (Foa & Kozak, 1986; Salkovskis, 1991), and that exposure also provides opportunities for spontaneous cognitive change (Jaycox, 1998). Careful examination of the cognitions, together with formulation, prepares the way for behavioral experiments tailored to the patient's own concerns, which may expedite treatment (see Chapters 2, 5, and 6).

Key Maintaining Processes

- Anxious predictions, based on exaggerated estimates of harm or danger, and underestimates of ability to cope or be rescued.
- Associated physiological arousal.
- Biased attention to phobic stimuli, and for bodily signs of anxiety that can fuel "fear of fear" (Rachman & Brichard, 1988) and may ultimately lead to a panic attack.
- Safety behaviors and avoidance that deny people the chance to test their beliefs.

Treatment Strategies

- Exposure to phobic objects, while directing attention toward processing the real object (rather than an image of it).
- Dropping safety behaviors and testing the consequences.
- At the same time observing the effects of the fear, and testing catastrophic predictions about this (e.g., "I will die or go mad if I get frightened").

Common Complicating Factors

Using the above strategies is frequently very efficacious in the treatment of specific phobias. However, phobias may coexist with other anxiety disorders, including panic disorder, OCD, posttraumatic stress disorder (PTSD), health anxiety, or depression. It is quite common for phobic patients to have panic cognitions, such as "I will die of fright," "My anxiety will never drop," "I will go crazy," and so on. Such cognitions can be challenged and tested, as they would be in panic disorder. Care must also be taken to ensure that the person really engages with the phobic situation, rather than employing subtle avoidance strategies or safety behaviors during treatment sessions that result in predictions not being properly tested.

A study by Pratt, Cooper, and Hackmann (2004) suggests that for some patients with simple phobias asking about images reveals important appraisals linked to negative core beliefs, and to upsetting early memories relevant to the onset of the phobia.

This may provide important material for the conceptualization and help with engagement, in that persons may then realize that they are being "haunted by a ghost from the past" and their phobia thus makes sense (see Chapter 2). Images can be deliberately updated by comparing them against present reality, utilizing behavioral experiments (Chapter 6). In addition it may be relevant to work on key early memories and associated core beliefs (Chapter 5).

Obsessive–Compulsive Disorder

The diagnostic criteria for OCD include obsessions (recurrent intrusive images, impulses or thoughts that are not simply excessive worries about real problems) and/or compulsions (repetitive behaviors that the person feels driven to perform in response to an obsession, or to rigid rules). The person attempts to ignore, suppress, or neutralize obsessions and recognizes that they are a product of their own mind. The compulsive behavior is aimed at reducing distress or preventing a dreaded outcome but is not connected in a realistic way with what it is designed to prevent, or is clearly excessive.

A Cognitive Understanding of OCD

Several cognitive models exist. Salkovskis (1985) suggested that obsessional intrusive thoughts and images begin as normal intrusions but are appraised as more threatening, and personally relevant. People with OCD see themselves as having power that is pivotal in bringing about or preventing negative outcomes and fear that they may be responsible for harm. Neutralizing behavior of various kinds is intended to reduce discomfort resulting from these faulty appraisals. Wells (1997) also stressed the importance of appraisals of intrusions and emphasized the role of attentional strategies. Freeston, Rheaume, and Ladouceur (1996) did acknowledge the importance of a sense of responsibility but also highlighted overestimation of threat, intolerance of uncertainty, and perfectionism.

A working group was set up with the aim of developing a possible consensus and further development of the models (OCCWG, 1997). Important belief domains in OCD are thought to include thought-action fusion, an inflated sense of responsibility, beliefs about the controllability of thoughts, perfectionism, overestimation of threat, and intolerance of uncertainty. The term "thought–action fusion" refers to the belief that thinking a "bad" thought can cause a bad consequence, or that thinking a bad thought is morally equivalent to carrying out a bad action (Shafran, Thordarson, & Rachman, 1996).

Key Maintaining Processes

- Overestimation of threat of danger and exaggerated sense of responsibility for harm.
- Intolerance of uncertainty, again linked to exaggerated sense of responsibility.
- Biased attention to cues signaling potential for harm.
- Checking for signs of harm (mistakes, contamination, etc.).
- Reassurance seeking.
- Safety behaviors and avoidance.

- Recurrent worry or rumination.
- Metacognitive beliefs of several kinds, such as thought-action fusion, which signify that appraisals must be acted upon, or harm will be caused. Also overestimation of the importance of thoughts, and the need to control them.

Treatment Strategies

- Patients are encouraged to test Theory 2 ("This is an anxiety problem") rather that Theory 1 ("The harm I fear is real"). As in health anxiety, this step is quite crucial for engagement (see Chapter 4).
- Careful assessment of appraisals is made, including the downward arrow to identify the "hot" appraisals that are typically avoided. Such appraisals answer questions about what the consequences of adverse outcomes might be (see Chapter 2).
- A variety of techniques including guided discovery, psychoeducation, and behavioral experiments are used to challenge the various belief domains that are relevant for each person. These domains include responsibility appraisals, overimportance of thought, need to control thoughts, overestimation of threat, intolerance of anxiety, and perfectionism.
- Patients are encouraged to carry out behavioral experiments to check whether their safety behaviors are counterproductive, and are actually maintaining the sense of fear.
- Behavioral experiments and guided discovery are used to discover how realistic the predictions of danger are, but this is not the main platform of treatment.

For fuller descriptions of treatment, see Morrison and Westbrook (2004); Salkovskis, Forrester, Richards, and Morrison (1999); Simos (2002); and Wells (1997).

Common Complicating Factors

There is extensive overlap between health anxiety, depression, social anxiety, low self-esteem and OCD. There is also a degree of comorbidity with PTSD. Studies have shown that in some cases a diagnosis of PTSD has preceded that of OCD (de Silva & Marks, 1999), and in a significant number of cases imagery in OCD consists of intrusive memories, whereas in many other cases the content of images is similar but not identical to disturbing memories (Speckens, Hackmann, & Ehlers, 2003).

Other complications are that some beliefs are close to being delusional in their intensity. Patients may also be reluctant to talk about (or even think about) the contents of their obsessional thoughts and images, preferring to keep them rather general and out of awareness, to avoid the associated affect. For some the feared outcomes may not be clear, or they lie in the far future (as in health anxiety), making them hard to test. Patients may find it hard to tolerate any degree of uncertainty or anxiety (Freeston et al., 1996).

Cognitive avoidance may need to be addressed, and the patient may need to learn to live with a degree of uncertainty (see Chapters 7 and 9). They may need to work on low self-esteem (see Chapter 8). The role of past traumatic experiences should be considered, and work on images and memories may be useful (see Chapter 5).

Generalized Anxiety Disorder

GAD is defined as excessive anxiety and worry (apprehensive expectation), occurring more days than not for a period of at least 6 months, about a number of events or activities. The disorder is defined in terms of a cognitive process: worry, of a minimum severity level to distinguish it from normal worry. Worry is perceived as difficult to control, leads to significant distress or impairment, and must be associated with at least three of six anxiety symptoms. It should not be due to another psychological, physiological, or medical condition.

A Cognitive Understanding of GAD

Three main models of GAD currently contribute to our understanding of the problem (Heimberg, Turk, & Mennin, 2004). Borkovec suggests that worry about past and future events is central to GAD, and although none of these events is occurring in the present, patients react as if they are currently threatened or at risk. Borkovec and Newman (1998) further suggest that worry is the product of attempts to avoid more acute distress, occasioned for example by disturbing imagery in the face of threat. Worrying has however been shown to interfere with emotional processing and reduces flexibility of responses.

Another model developed in Quebec, Canada (see Ladouceur et al., 2000) suggests that people with GAD find it very hard to tolerate uncertainty. They are reluctant to give threatening material their full attention and are slow to initiate problem solving (although once engaged in the process their performance may show no deficits). Worrying instead of fully engaging with the material may be a counterproductive strategy.

The metacognitive model of Wells (2000, 2002) distinguishes two types of worry in GAD. The first type (about potential threats) is triggered by mistaken beliefs about the usefulness of worry. The second type focuses on the potential negative effects of worry (e.g., "Worrying will drive me crazy"). Patients often report both types of belief and therefore find worry difficult to terminate, while being afraid of its effects.

Key cognitive themes include intolerance of uncertainty, fears of wide range of possible dangers, fear of being unable to cope with them, beliefs about the possible consequences of worrying, and underlying beliefs revealing a sense of vulnerability and inadequacy.

Key Maintaining Processes

- Wells (2000, 2002) described positive and negative beliefs about worry as metacognitive beliefs and highlighted the importance of both in GAD.
- The Quebec group suggests that patients with GAD are reluctant to give threatening material their full attention (e.g., Dugas et al., 1998) and Borkovec's group would endorse this (e.g., Borkovec & Newman, 1998).
- Worrying feels like thinking things through but may actually interfere with emotional processing (see Chapter 5) and problem solving.

Treatment Strategies

- In GAD the aim is to enhance tolerance for uncertainty and increase curiosity and flexibility because it is impossible to avoid all risks in life. Therapists are ill advised to start by directly challenging the patient's thoughts about bad things that might happen. By definition, there will be a large and shifting number of such concerns.

- Instead, there is a focus on metacognitive beliefs (positive and negative) about worry, and these can be challenged using guided discovery and behavioral experiments (Butler & Rouf, 2004).
- Other implications from the theories described above would be that patients should be encouraged to face and reflect on their disturbing images, memories, and thoughts rather than worrying excessively, so that "emotional processing" can occur (see Chapter 5).
- In addition, they can be encouraged to engage in problem solving in matters of more immediate concern, and distract themselves from those that have a low probability of occurring in the distant future.

Common Complicating Factors

Two-thirds of patients with GAD would describe themselves as "having always been a worrier," and dependent and avoidant personality characteristics are common. There is significant comorbidity with social anxiety, severe depression, and hopelessness, and low self-esteem is pervasive. There may be intolerance of any degree of uncertainty. A large proportion of patients with GAD report that at an early age they found themselves in situations that threatened to overwhelm them, such as having to cope with sick, absent, or alcoholic parents (Roemer, Borkovec, Posa, & Lyonfields, 1991). During therapy, worries presented may be vague, and patients may feel reluctant to disclose their true concerns.

Thus, avoidance of affect may need to be tackled (see Chapter 8), and patients may need encouragement to face, elaborate, and contextualize their frightening images and memories rather than worrying (Chapter 5). They may need help in learning to live with uncertainty, and their confidence and self-esteem may need to be enhanced during therapy (Chapters 6 and 9).

Posttraumatic Stress Disorder (PTSD)

DSM-IV-TR defines PTSD as a reaction to a profoundly distressing event that threatened death or serious injury to the self or others. The patient's response must have involved intense fear, helplessness, or horror. Key symptoms involve reexperiencing, avoidance, and hyperarousal.

A Cognitive Understanding of PTSD

The most comprehensive cognitive model (Ehlers & Clark, 2000) incorporates facets observed by many earlier authors. It is suggested that PTSD arises if the individual processes the traumatic event in a way that generates a sense of current threat. Two processes are postulated to create this perception: (1) excessively negative appraisals of the trauma and its consequences and (2) a disturbance of autobiographical memory characterized by strong perceptual memories that are affect laden and disconnected from their context. Unhelpful cognitive and behavioral strategies, including rumination, suppression of memories, avoidance, and hypervigilance maintain the problem.

Important cognitive themes include unhelpful appraisals of trauma consequences (PTSD symptoms, altered circumstances, losses, etc.) and negative appraisals of the traumatic event. The latter may involve the intensification of pretrauma beliefs, or the shattering of previous positive beliefs (Janoff-Bulman, 1992). There may also be distorted appraisals of the traumatic event, which are not updated even in the face of contradictory information. Any of the above themes can involve appraisals of the self, the world, or other people.

Key Maintaining Factors

- The nature of trauma memory appears to be crucial (Brewin, 2001; Ehlers & Clark, 2000). Trauma memories appear to be vivid, distressing sensory fragments of real (or imagined) parts of the trauma, stored without a time code, and without reference to other autobiographical information.
- Perceptual priming and associative learning mean that memory fragments and affect are easily and automatically triggered by low-level sensory cues, often without awareness of the trigger.
- Rumination appears to be another important maintenance factor.
- Hypervigilance and biased attention to danger are pronounced.
- There is usually extensive avoidance and a plethora of safety behaviors.

Treatment Strategies

- Reliving together with the downward arrow technique helps access all the meanings given to the traumatic event, which affected the way it was processed at the time and subsequently.
- Meaning is considered to be central, and the generation of alternative, more helpful perspectives seems at least as important as processes of habituation or extinction. An important procedure involves updating "hot spots" using verbal and imagery techniques (Ehlers, Clark, Hackmann, McManus, & Fennell, 2005; Grey, Young, & Holmes, 2002). For a detailed description, see Chapter 5.
- Attentional processes are targeted, and patients are encouraged to decrease their hypervigilance for danger but also learn to discriminate between what is actually happening now, and what is input from the traumatic memory.
- The overgeneralized sense of threat is explored and challenged, using behavioral experiments (Ehlers et al., 2005).

Because of the complexity of the phenomenology in PTSD only parts of the model are tackled at any one time, with vicious circles used to explain maintenance of each aspect of the problem. The therapist needs to utilize an array of procedures, with the order and prominence of strategies personalized for each case.

Common Complicating Factors

PTSD is an interesting disorder to treat, as patients can present with virtually any elements of the other anxiety disorders, or other Axis I or Axis II disorders. Sixty percent of patients with a primary diagnosis of PTSD meet criteria for at least one other disorder, most commonly depression (Kessler, Sonnega, Bromet, Hughes, & Nelson, 1995). Panic disorder and GAD are common, and patients may suffer from substance abuse or dependence, pain or disability caused by the trauma, and sometimes associated bereavements. Some patients also develop OCD (de Silva & Marks, 1999). Thus conceptualization needs to be very clear and focused, while incorporating all the relevant strands (see Chapter 2).

Attention must also be paid to the meanings given to the sequelae of the trauma (pain, disability, bereavement, financial and legal matters, etc.). Occasionally schema change methods are used when previous negative beliefs have been intensified. Sometimes it may be necessary to work on traumatic memories from earlier in the patient's life, where similar thematic content has caused various memories to bleed into each other (see Chapter 5).

Bearing all the strands in mind, and deciding what to target, can be a complex business. Formulation is an important key to an efficient and comprehensive approach within a limited time frame (see Chapter 2). Cognitive avoidance, and avoidance of affect, may present obstacles to successful treatment. Chronic low self-esteem can also complicate the picture (see Chapters 6 and 8).

EMBRACING COMPLEXITY WHILE UTILIZING SPECIFIC PROTOCOLS

It will already be apparent to the reader that, in the case of models and treatments for anxiety disorders, "specific" does not mean simple minded. Cognitive understanding of each disorder is sophisticated, and treatment strategies have been carefully tailored to target key cognitive processes. In many cases the outcome data from treatment trials has been outstanding.

However, a number of potential complicating factors emerge from consideration of the disorders described above. These include comorbidity; idiosyncratic underlying beliefs; distal factors and disturbances of memory; cognitive avoidance; avoidance of affect, intolerance of uncertainty; and low self-esteem. When the treatment is not progressing, reformulating the case and attending to one or more of these complicating factors can make the difference.

Comorbidity

The National Comorbidity Survey (Kessler et al., 1994) considered people with a number of Axis I and Axis II diagnoses, including panic disorder, agoraphobia, social phobia, simple phobia, and GAD. They found that about 60% of their sample had met criteria for three or more of the diagnoses within the previous 12-month period. For efficient treatment, conceptualization needs to be clear, focused, and capable of being shared with the patient, while still embracing complexity. In addition, decisions need to be made about how to interweave aspects of treatment from various specific models in any particular case. Knowledge of the developmental and maintaining processes highlighted by the specific models is a central element of this work. It helps the therapist to identify with precision the nature of the patient's anxieties, and to use this precision as a basis for a formulation that can integrate anxiety with other comorbid conditions.

In Chapters 2 and 3 we offer strategies for how to go about exploring key appraisals and developing useful formulations in straightforward as well as complicated cases involving anxiety. Chapter 4 explores how the formulation as well as other aspects of therapy can cultivate metacognitive awareness in complex cases—a necessary context for change. Chapter 8 addresses anxiety comorbid with depression.

Idiosyncratic Beliefs and Experience

Even if we start from what seems to be a DSM-IV-TR diagnosis of one specific anxiety disorder, we always need to ensure that we have not overlooked idiosyncratic aspects of the patient's experience. This can happen when we are too narrowly focused on "typical" cognitive themes and processes. There is a danger that rigidly applying a specific model or protocol for treatment might act like a schema for the therapist: Only information that fits with that model would be seen as a suitable target for treatment, while other data might be ignored, discounted, distorted or viewed as irrelevant.

In Chapter 2 we discuss how to counter this. Sharply focusing on emotionally "hot" material can lead to in-depth exploration of the most personally salient appraisals.

Distal Factors and Disturbances in Autobiographical Memory

Distal aspects of problems (their origins) are sometimes ignored in the treatment of anxiety disorders because so much "mileage" is usually achieved by focusing on (proximal) maintenance factors. The role of disturbances in autobiographical memory is clear in PTSD: It may also play a part in the other anxiety disorders, and similar treatment procedures may be useful. This is a suitable topic for research, and an area to explore in clinical practice.

Chapter 2 describes ways of exploring cognitions in depth, so that the appraisals that really drive the problem are identified and tackled in a systematic and comprehensive manner. This chapter draws on recent work on traumatic memories and their relationship to imagery and looks at the interpersonal dimensions of anxiety disorders, including fears about coping and rescue.

Chapter 5 covers working with images, metaphor, and memories that carry important meanings: convincing the heart as well as the head. This chapter builds on ideas discussed earlier, on new research on imagery and traumatic memories. Methods of updating memories across the anxiety disorders are described. The use of metaphor in cognitive therapy for anxiety disorders is explored.

Cognitive Avoidance and Avoidance of Affect

It can be difficult to tackle anxiety disorders without considering their context and relationship to other patient problems. Cognitive avoidance and avoidance of affect can make the treatment of any disorder difficult and may require particular attention. They can lead to a lack of specificity about events and their meanings, and to reluctance to address them, either in discussion or through behavioral experiments.

Methods of enhancing metacognitive awareness can help with cognitive avoidance. Patients learn that their thoughts are not facts and their images may not reflect reality. These are especially useful when anxiety is long-standing, or part of a more complex picture. In such cases patients may see taking steps to change things as risky at best, and impossible at worst, and find it difficult to achieve the distance from their own thinking that they need to engage effectively in treatment. We discuss this strategy in Chapter 4.

In Chapter 7 we will discuss how to overcome emotional avoidance, so that one can approach the heart of the matter and engage in effective cognitive-emotional processing. This is a problem that can occur in any anxiety disorder and is a defining feature of avoidant personality disorder.

Intolerance of Uncertainty

Intolerance of uncertainty can also bedevil treatment, particularly of GAD, health anxiety, and OCD. Chapter 9 discusses how to help patients to live with a certain amount of uncertainty, rather than attempting to obliterate anxiety completely, which is unrealistic for clinicians as well as patients.

Low Self-Esteem

Readers may have noted earlier that low self-esteem was implicated in the development and persistence of anxiety disorders right across the spectrum as well as in comorbidity with depression and substance abuse. Low self-esteem can undermine treatment of any anxiety disorder. Treatment often needs not only to combat anxiety but also to reduce depression and hopelessness. Chapter 8 presents a cognitive model of low self-esteem and shows how anxiety can be understood and worked with in a broader context of negative beliefs about the self.

Maintaining the Gains

Finally, in Chapter 10 we discuss how to ensure that patients have the tools they need to deal with future setbacks or other emotional problems. One strategy is to create a written blueprint for the patient. It provides a framework for patients to reflect on what has been achieved in therapy, and to use new learning as a basis for tackling future difficulties effectively.

CONCLUSION

As authors we draw on a wealth of clinical and research experience. Our attempts to apply the models (even with selected patients in research treatment trials) have led to refinements and elaboration of aspects of clinical practice, together with attempts to attend to some of the (complex) processes described above, enabling us to make sophisticated analyses of the best sequencing and combination of interventions in each case.

This chapter concludes with a vignette, to demonstrate the way in which elements of models for several disorders can be interwoven, and linked with material from the past.

A Clinical Vignette: Tackling Comorbidity

John was traveling home from work one day when his car was hit by a moving van with a heavy load. He presented with PTSD following this serious (unavoidable) traffic accident. He had lost confidence in his ability to drive and suffered from nightmares, flashbacks, and depression. He had tried very hard to hide these symptoms and had given other people the impression that his accident had been quite trivial, whereas at the time he was certain that he would die. This concealment and reluctance to involve others arose from his disturbed childhood about which he had also never spoken: his stepfather and his mother were neglectful, and his much older stepbrothers were very violent, so he had quickly learned that he should fend for himself. He had struggled on for months, fearing that he might be going mad, and contemplating suicide, before presenting for treatment.

Treatment for John's PTSD was proceeding quite well, and included *reliving and updating the memory of the car crash* (see Chapter 5), and some *in-vivo* driving practice on busy roads. However, John had had trouble making himself drive on wide roads. If he did, he immediately felt as if he was very tiny, and the road was huge; so big that he could get lost in it. This feeling was slightly reduced when he invented his own *behavioral experiment*, running straight across the road, and realizing more fully that he was a large adult, and the road was only about 12 feet wide.

However, he still felt afraid of fainting or losing control of the car he was driving. He was overbreathing and feeling very dizzy, and avoiding all but the smallest roads. The therapist tried some cognitive therapy for *panic*, including a series of *behavioral experiments*. First, the patient overbreathed briefly, discovering that this caused the symptoms that he was scared of, without making him faint. The therapist then encouraged him to do it for much longer, and did it herself. The intention behind this work on panic attacks was to prove to him that such symptoms do not ultimately lead to fainting or losing control of the body. However, though the therapist could still easily walk around, the patient froze and was unable to hear or talk to the therapist. The symptoms had activated a flashback of the crash. In addition, he linked his "freeze" reaction to how he had responded as a child, when he would assume the fetal position when hit by his stepbrothers. In other words, the *PTSD, panic disorder, and childhood memories were intertwined*. Discovering this was useful, and the patient practiced overbreathing, but staying grounded in the here and now, moving around rather than freezing, and reminding himself that he was an adult and no longer in danger.

Back on even bigger roads, his perception changed again: He was tiny, and out of control, not knowing where he was in space. The therapist investigated this further, asking when in his life he could remember feeling like that, and he immediately said that this "felt sense" was the same as he had had as a small child, when his stepbrothers would knock him around, bouncing him off the walls and the furniture. The therapist then got him to *rescript the memory*, visiting his little self, and removing and protecting him (see Chapter 5). The technique was borrowed from Axis II work (Arntz & Weertman, 1999; Weertman & Arntz, 2007). Subsequently he was able to retain the sense of himself as a large adult on a normal road when he was out driving. In addition, his recurrent nightmares of being a tiny person, out of control, and bounced around inside a huge car that he could not control disappeared after he had *rescripted his nightmares*, writing them out with different endings.

Thus in this case elements of the PTSD and the panic protocols were used, together with work on updating a traumatic childhood memory, more typical of Axis II work. All these strands were woven together.

PART II

DEEPENING UNDERSTANDING AND SECURING ENGAGEMENT

"I can't make it out. All of a sudden I'm in a panic, right out of the blue."
"None of it makes any sense. It's just one big mess."
"It's not how it looks, *it's how it* is."

These three comments from patients illustrate difficulties that commonly emerge in the early stages of cognitive therapy. Each has the potential to prevent patients fully engaging in the process of change, whereas identifying and resolving them opens the door to emotional transformation. Ideas about how to recognize these difficulties as well as about how to overcome them are presented in the following three chapters.

The first comment above illustrates the importance of careful assessment in illuminating cognitive processes that may occur so swiftly, and with such emotional force, that patients have difficulty identifying them clearly. The second highlights the value of case formulation, not merely in mapping the territory of the problem, but also in helping patients to gain a sense that their problems have an underlying logic, and that practical solutions to them can be found. The third illustrates a common feature of anxiety, especially when affect is high and physical arousal at a pitch—patients' difficulty in seeing that their perspective, even though it feels objectively real, may be just one of many possible views, and perhaps not the most realistic or helpful. All of these difficulties can impede the process of engagement in cognitive therapy, and resolving them thus forms a crucial step toward active change.

In Chapter 2, "Assessment: Investigating Appraisals in Depth," we address the central issue of accurately identifying idiosyncratic, emotionally charged cognitions central to the experience of anxiety, whether these take the form of words, images, memories, or a "felt sense." Only through careful assessment of these can treatment be precisely targeted. In Chapter 3, "Case Formulation: Making Sense of Complexity," we move on to consider how information gathered during the assessment process forms the basis for coherent, theoretically driven, tailor-made case formulations. These permit us to conceptualize predisposing, precipitating, and maintaining factors, even in complex, multifaceted cases of anxiety with long histories and high comorbidity, where the basic disorder-specific models may be of limited use. In Chapter 4, "Decentering from Thoughts: Achieving Objectivity," we show how collaboratively mapping processes central to the maintenance of anxiety can help patients to achieve "metacognitive awareness." That is, they come to understand that their beliefs, however compelling, are just ideas learned through experience, which they can choose to question and test, accept or reject.

TWO

Assessment
Investigating Appraisals in Depth

This chapter starts from the assumption that accurate assessment of cognitions, at deeper as well as at more superficial levels, is essential for effective treatment. It is especially important when progress does not proceed as, supposedly, it should. In this chapter we consider a wide range of methods for identifying appraisals in cognitive therapy. As we discussed in the Preface, cognitive models of the anxiety disorders largely and usefully focus on maintaining factors that are relatively disorder specific, such as catastrophic misinterpretation of bodily sensations in panic, and fear of negative evaluation in social phobia. One of the great strengths of the disorder-specific models is that they encourage us to focus down on particular patterns of cognition and behavior. This emphasis is extremely illuminating, and it often helps the therapist to anticipate the content of a patient's thoughts. However, it may also mean that relevant, idiosyncratic meanings are missed in a particular case. Even within a specific diagnostic category each patient's experience, appraisal of that experience, and pattern of response is unique.

Idiosyncratic appraisals may be driving unusual safety behaviors, and thus maintaining the problem. Sharpening the focus on appraisals through careful assessment sets the scene for better formulation, which paves the way for more informative behavioral experiments and gives the patient the framework for understanding that input from the past may be coloring their view of the present. When atypical or multiple cognitive factors make it hard to apply a standard protocol, then developing a shared and detailed understanding of the patient's "felt sense" in difficult situations also assists with engagement.

Of course, assessment of cognitions comes in the context of a full assessment carried out using all the usual methods, and attending to the processes involved in building a therapeutic, open, and collaborative relationship. These methods, and others preliminary to starting a course of cognitive-behavioral treatment such as explaining the cognitive model and the active role expected of the patient, eliciting expectations for therapy, and modeling a structured approach to resolving psychological difficulties by using clear agenda setting, frequent feedback, and summaries, are well described elsewhere.

Here we consider ways of looking at appraisals carried by images, memories, metaphors, dreams, and more nebulous feelings in the body, as well as the classic, mainly verbal methods of examining cognitions. We make a distinction between the "propositional" or analytical level of meaning, and the more "implicational" level of meaning accompanied by emotion, which may be harder to put into words (Barnard & Teasdale, 1991). We trace links between the "felt sense" of danger and its possible historical roots. This chapter on assessment of meaning is intended to prepare the ground for Chapters 5 and 6, in which we look at a wide range of powerful methods for transforming meaning that are particularly useful when working with complex or atypical cases. But, of course, it also plays an essential part in providing information for the work of formulation described in the next chapter.

STANDARD METHODS OF ACCESSING APPRAISALS

As discussed in Chapter 1, Beck's (e.g., Beck, 1976) theory postulates that emotional disturbance is triggered by appraisals, including thoughts and images, which are accessible via the contents of consciousness. Affect is considered to be an important "marker" that indicates the presence of relevant appraisals. Standard texts give extensive guidance on how to access and examine this material, particularly using verbal techniques (e.g., J. S. Beck, 1995; Beck et al., 1979, 1985; Leahy, 2003; Padesky & Greenberger, 1995; Wells, 1997; Westbrook & Kirk, 2007). Four classic methods are briefly summarized here, before the topic is given wider consideration.

First, there is a consensus that it is important to examine "hot" material, that is, those meanings that are present when affective disturbance is marked. Emphasis is placed on uncovering appraisals that are strong enough to account for the feelings aroused. Patients may fear external or internal events (being involved in a traffic accident, or imagining such an event). In addition, they may fear negative—or even disastrous—effects of the presence (or absence) of particular thoughts, images, memories, bodily sensations, or associated affect (being rejected because of profuse sweating, or being unable to remember how to perform simple tasks at work).

Second, anxiety is considered to be a product of a combination of factors: the person's perception of the likelihood of a feared outcome, its awfulness, available resources for coping with it, and any possible rescue factors (Beck et al., 1985). Therefore it is important for therapists to explore all aspects of what has been called the *anxiety equation*:

$$\text{Anxiety is a function of: } \frac{\text{Probability} \times \text{Cost of feared event}}{\text{Coping} + \text{Rescue factors}}$$

Third, upsetting appraisals can be more closely examined by using the *downward arrow* technique. If the patient describes a distressing event but ascribes a meaning to it that does not seem to account for the apparent distress, the therapist can ask "and what was the worst thing about that?" This can be repeated several times, with the patient usually describing more distressing, idiosyncratic meanings at each stage. This procedure very quickly evokes affect and higher order meanings.

Finally, a study of *emerging themes and generalities* can provide clues to the patient's relevant core beliefs and assumptions. These then become therapy targets as treatment progresses.

TARGETING HIGHER LEVEL APPRAISALS

This next section places these standard techniques in the wider context of multilevel models of cognitive processing. As we show, there are links between the patient's current phenomenology and autobiographical memory. This discussion then leads to practical suggestions for how to prepare the ground and access the type of material that will allow precise targeting of appraisals in anxiety across disorders, including complex cases with extensive comorbidity.

Examining Cognitions When Affect Is High

It has been suggested that when affect is high, not only is it easier to access higher order meanings, but also challenging cognitions at this point may produce more profound change than that which is achieved by discussing the material more dispassionately. This key hypothesis requires some exploration.

The notion of "dual belief systems" was elaborated in relation to anxiety disorders by Beck and colleagues (1985) and refers to the observation that it is possible for an anxious person to have two sets of contradictory beliefs about a situation. Well away from danger, the estimated probability of a catastrophe may seem very small, but as proximity increases it rises dramatically, and "hot" cognitions and affect emerge. For example, the plane has a low probability of crashing when you book the flight, but a crash feels certain at the point of departure.

Beck and colleagues (1985) also noted that, in addition to triggering negative automatic thoughts and anxiety, approaching the feared situation can trigger visual and somatic imagery, so that the anxious person begins to experience in fantasy the catastrophic consequences he or she fears. For example, Beck and colleagues described a person with a height phobia who experienced the floor tilting away from her at a steep angle in a skyscraper, and a man who, fearing a heart attack, experienced chest pains when far from medical help. Clearly in these examples the term "imagery" is used to describe a mental representation of something, not by direct observation but by memory or imagination, and the content need not be exclusively visual.

Borkovec (2004) described something similar. He observed that when people worry about terrible things that might happen they react as if the disaster has already occurred, even though they "know" it has not. The idea that there may be two different types of cognitive processing (in broad terms consisting either of thoughts or of imagery) has a long history. For a review see Power (1997), who suggested that this hypothesis was even advanced by Freud and by Janet, at the end of the 19th century.

Examining the Whole "Felt Sense"

When affect is high the contents of consciousness are likely to be mixed and contribute to what Gendlin (1996) called the "felt sense." Verbal thoughts may be interspersed

with imagery, while emotions and other bodily sensations are also present. Interestingly, cognitive therapists rarely inquire about bodily sensations, although these can be
quite informative. For example, patients with PTSD often reexperience physical sensations they had at the time of the trauma (Rothschild, 2000; van der Kolk, 1994). These
are not exclusively the sensations of emotion but may include what appears to be input
from memory, such as pain or crushing sensations (after a car crash), heat (after a fire),
or extreme coldness (after almost drowning). Such sensations can be triggered by certain sensory cues reminiscent of the trauma. Similarly, in the other anxiety disorders
body sensations can echo past upsetting experiences, as was the case for Colin, whose
experiences during panic attacks were linked to memories of childhood.

> Colin was suffering from panic attacks. Reading or thinking about death could
> trigger these. In each attack he imagined himself trapped in a box, unable to ever
> get out. He could see nothing but blackness, but felt his limbs constricted and
> heard the sound of his own heart pounding. He had the sense that after his death
> he would find himself trapped in a box as a form of punishment. Colin had had
> these ideas about death since he was a small boy. His father had locked him in a
> small cupboard for hours at a stretch and left him there in the dark. He had lived
> next to a graveyard, had seen coffins being buried, and had vividly imagined peo-
> ple feeling trapped inside and all alone.

In some types of therapy patients are encouraged to focus on how an upsetting
experience reverberates in the body, and to elicit metaphors for how this feels. This is
one way of starting to explore meanings or appraisals underpinning the experience,
and their possible history (Gendlin, 1996; Greenberg & Paivio, 1997). Such methods can
be incorporated into cognitive therapy and may be useful in complex cases to explore
the phenomenology, the appraisals that are activated, and the history of this "felt
sense." This process is well articulated by Layden, Newman, Freeman, and Byers
Morse (1993). One of our own cases is described below.

> Judith met diagnostic criteria for borderline personality disorder (BPD) and found
> managing her emotions very difficult. She hated discussing emotional topics and
> constantly accused her therapist of "pushing her into the black," at which point the
> therapist tended to change the topic to calm her down. One day she asked Judith
> to just stay with the feeling and describe it. Judith said that everything was "going
> black," and she felt dizzy. She feared that if she stayed with the feeling she would
> become unconscious and would be annihilated. She then spontaneously connected
> this to experiences she had had as a little child, when her foster mother would
> leave her crying and screaming in her cot for what felt like hours. On several occa-
> sions this led to breath-holding attacks, and she had to be taken to hospital. The
> appraisals accessed by exploring this material included the belief that strong emo-
> tion could be life threatening, and that other people callously activated this quite
> deliberately. Both of these beliefs were identified and subsequently challenged in
> therapy.

An understanding of the ways in which input from memory of past distressing
events can color experiences in the present can help a patient gain a metacognitive per-

spective (as described in more detail in Chapter 4), and make it easier for them to start discriminating between what happened then, and what might really be happening now.

Imagery in the Anxiety Disorders

Recent studies of imagery in the anxiety disorders (many of which are presented in an extensive review by Holmes & Hackmann, 2004) suggest that distressing images can provide a wealth of information relevant to case conceptualization. These images can depict scenarios the patient fears and often flesh out aspects of the anxiety equation, such as the cost of the feared outcome, or the lack of support from others. They may graphically reveal information about core beliefs and assumptions that one might reach by using the downward arrow technique. For example, two people with panic disorder might fear fainting: Although the images of both might depict the likely interpersonal consequences of having a panic attack, the images could be quite different. One person might imagine a large crowd gathering and people laughing at them, while the other might have images of people walking by and totally ignoring his or her predicament. Such images might be accompanied by quite different emotions and safety behaviors. In addition, as in the cases of Judith and Colin, images may at first appear to be metaphorical rather than historical in content.

Wells (2000) proposed a special role for intrusive imagery. He suggested that it provides input from memory concerning cause and effect, and reveals appraisals of a situation and plans for meeting associated goals. In short, imagery can be one manifestation of a schema, with its constellations of interlinked cognitive, behavioral, physiological, and affective elements.

In a similar vein, Conway and colleagues (2004) suggested that some of the processes that drive human cognition and behavior cannot be brought directly into consciousness. Instead, the output of processes that occur out of awareness can be experienced as mental representations (including images) or actions. They suggest that spontaneous images are highly associated with goals and are close to actions. They also suggest that intrusive imagery depicts states of affairs that the person really wishes to avoid if at all possible. For example, an image of collapsing and being ignored might be associated with the goal of staying near to caring people, which then determines behavior. The implication is that reflecting on spontaneous imagery can be informative for patient and therapist by revealing the way in which the person is processing events and planning responses.

The idea of "dual belief systems" is also echoed in the work of Barnard and Teasdale (1991) who described two levels of meaning, in the context of their model of interacting cognitive subsystems (ICS). One is the propositional (shared, analytical) level of meaning, and the other is the implicational (idiosyncratic, holistic) level of meaning, which Teasdale asserted is the only level capable of directly producing emotion. Teasdale suggested that it is this idiosyncratic "felt sense" of things that should be activated and held in mindful awareness in therapy, while new, incompatible chunks of information are accumulated (Teasdale, 1999b). For example, at the propositional level we have a shared concept of a dog, whereas someone recently bitten by a fierce dog will have a rather different implicational-level representation. To restructure their implicational-level meaning of "dog" the person will need to have new experiences connected with dogs, while being in a fit state to process the fresh information provided.

This overview suggests that situational cues trigger more emotion and give access to more meanings associated with troublesome situations, than mere discussion. As Beck (e.g., 1976) suggested, these meanings are accessible through verbal thoughts, but also via imagery, which can be in any sensory modalities, especially the visual and somatic. Imagery can be closely linked to action, including avoidance and safety behaviors. It is also of interest that intrusive imagery often incorporates echoes from the past. It is to this topic that we now turn our attention.

INPUT FROM MEMORY IN THE ANXIETY DISORDERS

Beck (e.g., Beck et al., 1985, pp. 5, 210–213) has frequently noted that when affect is high, imagery involving memories or "reminiscence" may be part of the contents of consciousness. Several theorists have been curious about this and have speculated about the nature and functions of imagery and its links to memory (see Holmes & Hackmann, 2004).

In this section we first examine phenomenology in PTSD and then compare this with phenomenology in the other anxiety disorders. We begin with PTSD because much of the work on this topic originated from the study of this disorder. We refer to several relevant theoretical models that we believe may be applicable to the wide range of other anxiety disorders (and beyond). The theoretical ideas described in this section are relatively new and expand our ideas about key cognitive processes that may play a part across disorders. This may have important implications for assessment, formulation, and treatment.

Some Similarities Between Phenomenology in PTSD and in the Other Anxiety Disorders

PTSD is grouped with the anxiety disorders in DSM-IV-TR (APA, 2000) despite the fact that though anxiety disorders involve concern about current or future threat, PTSD centers on memory for a *past* distressing event. Ehlers and Clark (2000) suggested that one may resolve this puzzle by postulating that in PTSD the trauma has been processed in a way that signals *current* serious threat. Indeed, recurrent intrusive memories (which are triggered very readily by situational cues) do appear to signal current threat, in a way that often appears odd to patients, once they are away from the situation (exemplifying "dual belief systems"). In addition, the intrusive memories evoked often appear to be encoded and/or retrieved without their proper context or a time code. They appear disconnected from logic and from other autobiographical knowledge the person may possess, as in the following extraordinary example.

Fred was afraid to visit the hospital where his daughter had died several years ago, amidst a horrible family row. He thought he would find the memories very distressing. However, once he and the therapist reached the hospital he became afraid of potential events rather than memories. He feared that his brother (who lived abroad) might suddenly appear in the corridor again and shout at him, and he was also terrified of visiting the ward because he feared that his daughter would still be there in the hospital bed, although he had attended her funeral and therefore "knew" this could not be true.

In addition, input from memory can give rise to vivid and frightening images, without patients necessarily even being aware of the source of the input, or having any other contextual information to help them appreciate that the image is a memory fragment.

Jean had recurrent images at night of two staring eyes on a black background. She became frightened that this might be a ghost haunting her. However, her daughter inquired whether it could possibly be connected with a recent car crash. Immediately Jean realized that the image was identical to the approaching headlights she had seen on the night of the crash through her rearview mirror.

In PTSD it is also possible for affect and/or behavior to be triggered without the patient being aware of relevance of the situational cues.

Betty was having an MRI scan, following a car crash in which she had hurt her back. She suddenly felt extremely claustrophobic, fearing she would never get out, and started banging loudly on the righthand side of the cylinder. Reliving this episode later she realized that she had felt as if she was back in the car again after it had crashed, and was banging on the car door as she had done at the time, trying to get out before the car caught fire. The similar sensory aspects of the situation (i.e., being trapped within a metal device) had triggered the memory.

Sometimes in trauma memories there appears to be input from much earlier memories, as in the case of John (see also Chapter 1, p. 24), who experienced himself after a traffic accident in flashbacks and nightmares as a tiny little person in a huge vehicle over which he had no control, on a vast road. This appeared to incorporate material from memories of being physically abused, and knocked around as a very small child, bounced off the walls and furniture. The patient made this connection after describing the sensations he had had when his car was knocked across the road by a moving van with a heavy load, and he just managed to avoid hitting the center median by swerving back across the road.

In short "individuals with PTSD suffer inundation of images, sensations, and behavioral impulses ... disconnected from context, concepts and understanding" (Rothschild, 2000, p. 12).

Hackmann and Holmes (2004) argued that observations concerning spontaneous imagery in PTSD may have wider transdiagnostic applicability, particularly perhaps in anxiety disorders. Imagery across the other anxiety disorders also involves sensory intrusions, warning of potential distressing events. Much of it is recurrent, in a variety of modalities, and accompanied by strong affect. In addition, although the image signals *current* threat, much of the content appears to reflect input from earlier upsetting events, often without an immediate recognition by the individual that the source of threat is in the past, rather than the present. A review of the literature suggests striking parallels between phenomenology in PTSD and in anxiety in other Axis I, Axis II, and complex disorders with comorbidity. Just as in PTSD, some of the visual and somatic imagery anxious patients experience may consist of fragments of memory from earlier experiences, complete with their (nonupdated) meanings.

> Freda suffered from panic attacks and health anxiety. She had a recurrent somatic image during panic attacks of her soul leaving her body, and spiraling down toward Hell. She would repeatedly touch parts of her body and the furniture to check that her soul was still in her body. On reflection she thought that this experience was very like one she had as a child, when she had emergency surgery. Her parents had often taken her to a church where the priest preached extensively about Hell. As she lost consciousness during the anesthetic, and felt as if she was falling, she was afraid that her soul was leaving her body and was on the way to Hell.

Imagery in other anxiety disorders also often appears to consist of fragments of memory, which lack the contextual information that would make it obvious to the people that what they were experiencing was input from memory, rather than a warning of current danger.

> Jim had a snake phobia. He suffered from recurrent images of a snake chasing him at shoulder level, which he considered quite bizarre. However, he suddenly realized that when he was a small boy in Africa his brothers would hold harmless snakes at shoulder height and chase him around the garden, which was probably where the images came from.

Other clinicians have made similar observations. For example, Layden and colleagues (1993) described a patient with BPD, who was unaware until she was in therapy of fleeting images of her mother's face. These were triggered when the patient felt she was being rejected. The patient's mother had been severely depressed when the patient was 4 years old, and the images of her mother's passive, unresponsive face still triggered powerful emotions years later, without the patient being aware of their source. Sometimes behavior when the fear is activated can be quite informative, concerning the person's beliefs and their origins.

> Tom suffered from a wasp phobia. Confronted by a wasp he would invariably panic and cover his left ear. He commented that this was because a wasp had once flown into his ear and stung him, ushering in the phobia.

Layden and colleagues (1993) made a similar observation, in their description of another patient with BPD, who frequently became totally stone faced and numb during therapy sessions. Focusing on the felt sense at this point revealed that this occurred when the patient feared that someone cared for her, and then automatically numbed her own feelings. This response appeared to have arisen during sexual abuse from her stepbrother years before, and then became overgeneralized to all situations where she felt cared for by a man.

A study by Day, Holmes, and Hackmann (2004) on images and early memories in agoraphobia provides evidence of many cases in which there were apparent links between warning images of possible physical or mental catastrophes and their inter-personal consequences in the present, and distressing memories of separation, neglect, or lack of protection in the past. In many cases people were surprised that they had not considered these links before.

In some cases the imagery reported is recognized as a memory immediately. For example, in a study by Speckens and colleagues (2003) on OCD, two-thirds of the patients reported recurrent, intrusive imagery, and when asked if the image was actu-ally a memory many of the patients recognized them as such.

Upsetting images and memories help flesh out the details of the anxiety equation (i.e., how awful the feared event would be, and where the concerns lie in terms of potential coping and rescue factors). They may also provide material for the case for-mulation, if there are obvious links between the imagery, past upsetting events, and core beliefs and assumptions. Appraisals of intrusive images and memories can be an important maintenance factor. For example, if the patient interprets them as signaling current threat this can trigger associated safety behaviors.

Thus in anxiety disorders generally there are signs of incomplete emotional pro-cessing of past events, and contents of consciousness that are "Out of proportion, out of context, or simply out of time" (Rachman, 1980). This is a subject we return to in detail in Chapter 5.

Joan presented for treatment of agoraphobia, from which she had suffered for most of her adult life. She was also very anxious in social situations and had dependent and avoidant personality traits. She became demoralized extremely easily and felt depressed and hopeless after every panic attack. She avoided all social situations and found work extremely stressful, as it involved visiting unfamiliar places, where she feared she might get trapped or be taken ill.

The therapist decided to focus first on Joan's panic attacks. Every week she reported having several attacks, and these were reflected upon in detail, to access the catastrophic misinterpretations she was making, which were numerous. Her fears included fainting, having a stroke or a heart attack, having a brain tumor that might suddenly incapacitate her, going crazy, suddenly going blind, losing her memory, having an epileptic fit, and many more physical or mental problems. Behavioral experiments were carried out, during which she was encouraged to drop her safety behaviors, and then discover the true causes and consequences of her frightening symptoms. This met with scant success.

The therapist was becoming almost as disheartened as the patient. She then decided to inquire about imagery during a recent panic attack. The patient responded by reporting a recurrent frightening image, which almost always occurred in panic attacks. In it she collapsed and was taken to hospital against her will, where she remained trapped forever, and without visitors.

The therapist asked the patient to reflect upon whether she had ever had an experience like this in the past. The patient exclaimed that she suddenly realized where this image came from. As a little child she had frequently been told that she was unwanted, and her parents wished she had never been born. They lived in a very isolated place, and she felt very insecure. It was in this context that she had had a traumatic experience. She needed to have her tonsils out, and her parents took her to hospital. On arriving there she was put to bed, and her parents left, saying they would be back soon. However, they did not return for some days. Initially she concluded that she was lost, but the staff ignored her pleas to be taken home. On the second day she decided that her parents had found a way to get rid of her and were not coming back.

This was the source of the higher order meanings activated in adult life by the prospect of being taken ill in a place far from home. Interestingly, the patient had not previously made the connection between this childhood trauma and her felt sense during panic attacks. Once this connection had been made, therapy proceeded much more effectively because it had been possible to access other aspects of the anxiety equation, concerning the awfulness of being taken ill far from home, and her evaluation of her ability to cope or be rescued. Her panic attacks were driven by the fear that if she did become ill she would be trapped in a hostile place, unable to assert herself or get home, and that no one would help her. She feared that her current family would also not want her to return.

In this and a number of the other cases described above assessing the imagery and exploring its meanings and its relevance in the past and the present helped to resolve difficulties in therapy. It is important to note that the imagery reflects material that owes more to past than to present reality, and that it reveals incomplete processing of highly charged emotional events in the past. For further discussion of this matter, see Hackmann and colleagues (2000) on social phobia, Speckens and colleagues (2003) on OCD, Day and colleagues (2004) on agoraphobia, Pratt and colleagues (2004) on spider phobia, and Wells and Hackmann (1993) on health anxiety.

Theoretical Models with Potential Relevance to Memory in the Anxiety Disorders

The striking similarities between phenomenology in PTSD and the other anxiety disorders suggest that similar memory mechanisms may be involved. Several theorists have described and attempted to conceptualize the nature and significance of these memory features. We consider some of these briefly here, as this sets the scene for understanding the basis for methods of transforming meanings that we describe in Part III.

Ehlers and Clark (2000) discussed how in PTSD intrusive memory fragments intrude without a proper sense of their context among other memories. Despite being about the past they signal a real sense of *current* threat. Ehlers and colleagues (2002) noted that intrusive memories mainly reflect moments during the trauma when the meaning changed (usually for the worse). Excessively negative appraisals were often made at that time, and the intrusive memories with their associated warnings of danger tend to persist rather than be updated, even in the face of subsequent events that disconfirm these ideas.

Karen's two children died in a house fire. She had intrusions for many years after the fire of seeing the living room curtains ablaze and thinking her children might be in that room burning. The intrusions persisted, despite the fact that later she identified their bodies and observed that they were not burned but had been quickly overcome by fumes. Karen was amazed that the "horror fragments" of intrusive memory had persisted for many years and had not even connected with her own observations in the hospital.

Conway and colleagues (2004) described how memories are normally organized by themes (e.g., "houses I have lived in") or time periods (e.g., "when I was at school"), in a well-organized "filing system." This makes them easier to access deliberately, but also inhibits spontaneous triggering. However, during very upsetting experiences there may be extremely *negative self-defining moments* when personal goals are severely challenged. The theory suggests that such memories may not become part of the overall memory base and so may remain easily triggered. Because they have no "date-stamp" they can seem to signal current threat and hence prompt avoidance. This impedes the realization that the past is the past, the danger is no longer present, and these are only memory fragments that can be safely laid to rest.

The third theoretical framework, described by Brewin (Brewin, 2001; Brewin, Dalgleish, & Joseph, 1996) offers a cognitive-neuroscience account of the two kinds of memory following a traumatic event, with their different retrieval routes.

These three theoretical accounts of intrusive memories make the observation that upsetting sensory fragments of memory can be easily triggered. This appears to be true across many disorders. It appears that if overgeneralized negative meanings have been given to events, vivid sensory memories often lead to marked avoidance of these memories and their potential triggers. This makes it difficult for the remembered events to be contextualized among other memories, resulting in recurrent intrusions. We return to this topic, and to other ideas about emotional processing, in Chapter 5.

The relationship between excessively negative appraisals made during upsetting experiences and material intruding into consciousness (including memory fragments and other imagery), is illustrated in Figure 2.1, together with some typical responses that may maintain the problem. This diagram encapsulates the processes described above, and it can be simplified and adapted for use with individual patients, using their own idiosyncratic material. There are several examples of the use of this "vicious flower" model in Chapter 4.

HOW SHOULD WE ACCESS "HOT COGNITIONS"?

What is the best way to access these appraisals, that many people are at first not aware of, and that drive distress? First we discuss the context in which to carry out this work and then outline a number of methods for targeting and unpacking distorted appraisals.

Preparing the Ground

Accessing hot cognitions and higher order meanings in anxious people will understandably give rise to an increase in anxiety and possibly other emotions too. This means that careful preparation is important to maintain trust and preserve the therapeutic relationship. For example, patients are unlikely to relish the prospect of becoming very emotional in front of the therapist whom they do not know well. Nor will they

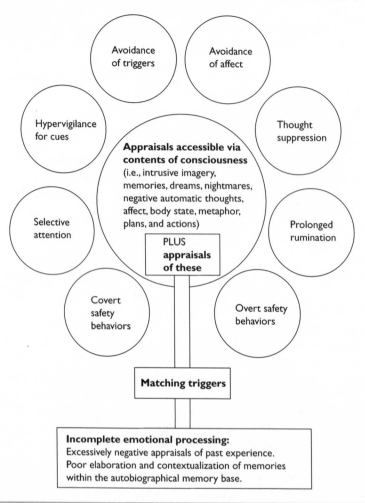

FIGURE 2.1. Model of origins and maintenance of negative appraisals in anxiety disorders.

be eager to share shameful memories (such as years of bullying in social phobia) without establishing trust.

Patients may be afraid that there will be a horrible outcome if they access hot material. They may fear insanity, unremitting anxiety, passing out, or even death. Some work on these cognitions may need to be undertaken in a compassionate manner before the session can proceed. Reassurance, normalization, and provision of information about the effects of anxiety can be helpful. Where there are fears of a real physical or mental catastrophe some cognitive therapy for panic, including relevant behavioral experiments, may be helpful, whatever the target anxiety disorder (Bennett-Levy, Butler, et al., 2004). If the material is too distressing to talk about it may be worth starting by asking the patient to write or draw instead, as this provides a "cooler" emotional space (Brewin & Lennard, 1999; Butler & Holmes, in press; and see also Chapter 7 on avoidance of affect). Finally, the therapist must be sure not to lead the patient, or be led by the patient's own imagination, rather than ensuring that the meaning comes from the patient.

Conversely, because of the dual belief systems outlined above, patients may in fact be quite unaware of just how upsetting it may be to approach material they have been strenuously avoiding. They may also have forgotten exquisitely distressing parts of highly emotional events, which may be retrieved in therapy. It is therefore important to pace the sessions appropriately, in case the patient becomes very distressed and has no time to recover or reflect on the meanings accessed by the end of the session. Adequate time must be budgeted for sessions involving exploring links with past traumatic experiences, reliving, situational exposure, or discussion of recent, specific examples of upsetting situations. Several sessions may be needed to arrive at a new perspective, and the patient needs to feel safe and grounded between the sessions. Examining images and memories in vivid detail can be like clicking on an icon and opening a computer file to reveal its full contents. This may initially be disturbing, but it is often a useful preparation for the work that needs to be done in therapy.

Finally the therapist's own clinical judgement must be used when deciding when or whether to ask the patient to relive very upsetting memories. Where there has been a history of repeated, prolonged, or very severe traumatization, particularly in childhood, many other therapeutic ingredients may need to be in place when and if this type of exploration is embarked upon. Trust and safety issues are paramount, and the patient should have his or her own grounding techniques and other resources in place first.

Eliciting "Hot" Material

An important focus of treatment not only in PTSD but also in other disorders is to examine moments when material from the past is activated in the present and distorts perception of events. Intrusive images and memories, arousal, affect, and safety behaviors are markers for distorted appraisals. Studies suggest that such material often maps closely onto "hot spots" in upsetting memories, carrying important meanings, and reflecting "negative self-defining moments" that threatened the person's sense of self and purpose (Conway et al., 2004). Such material can be brought "on line" by providing appropriate situational or imaginal cues, or by retrospectively examining events.

There are two main methods of accessing hot material. One is by recalling or imagining being in a feared situation and the other is by examining the "felt sense" when exposed to a feared situation. Most therapists begin by asking the patient to describe a recent, specific episode. Human beings possess imagination, and we know that imagery can evoke powerful affect. Specific memories may be more likely to be accompanied by affect and imagery than more-general memories (e.g., Mansell & Lam, 2004), confirming the suggestion that it may be useful to explore *specific* memories of particular events, rather than discuss problems in general terms. These memories may be of recent events, or of salient events long ago.

Accessing Cognitions by Recalling or Imagining a Specific Feared Situation

Cognitions are often explored by reflecting on a recent episode when the affect was high, and getting the patient to set the scene and describe it slowly, in very great detail. This is done to fully evoke a specific memory of the event. Usually more affect is evoked, and more detail revealed, than if instances of the problem are talked about more generally. This process uses imaginal cues to evoke hot material. Once this is activated various aspects can be explored. The patient can be asked about thoughts, imagery, body sensations, metaphors for the situation, and so on. The downward arrow technique can be used to ascertain information about the feared awfulness of the situation, and coping and rescue factors (or the lack of them). The material elicited is often highly idiosyncratic.

For example, during assessment for treatment of social phobia the patient is asked to describe a recent, specific example of the problem. A series of questions are asked about the situation, the thoughts the patient had about what might happen, what safety behaviors the patient began to apply, and where the patient's attention was focused. At this point the patient is asked whether he or she had an image or impression of how he or she might be coming across, or of how others might react to him or her. Almost all patients report a negative, distorted self- image, seen from an observer perspective, and also report that this image is typically recurrent. The images vary widely in content (Hackmann et al., 2000).

> One patient with social phobia reported feeling very small in a social situation, another reported seeing himself as a "nothing" and having an image of an empty chair where he should be, and a third saw himself as obese (which he was not at that time but had been as a teenager).

Making an "Emotional Bridge" to the Past

This technique (utilized in hypnotherapy, and sometimes called "the affect bridge"; Watkins, 1971) is also often used in cognitive therapy, particularly for providing a therapeutic focus in work with Axis II disorders (Beck, Freeman, & Associates, 1990; Layden et al., 1993; Young, Klosko, & Weishaar, 2003). However, it transpires that it is also useful in the examination of phenomenology in Axis I disorders and may be very productive in complex cases.

If detailed examination of situations that trigger anxiety reveals that the person has recurrent intrusive imagery, which seems to signal current threat, it may be useful to ask when the person first remembers having the sorts of thoughts, emotions, or sensory experiences that are reflected in the image. This often leads the person to realize that there may be more input from memory in the imagery than the person had previously appreciated, and that one or more traumatic experiences may be coloring the person's view of the present.

> Jane was being treated for social anxiety. Examination of episodes when she felt especially anxious revealed that she had a recurrent image of herself as hot and sweaty with rivers of sweat running down her face, even in cold weather. Her appraisals were: "I am a nervous wreck, a fraud. They will discover I know nothing." Inquiry as to when she had first had this distressing image led to the conclusion that its origin appeared to lie in events that occurred when she returned to a stressful job after both her parents had died suddenly. It was a very hot summer, and her boss's room was under the eaves of a tall, old building. The patient would

arrive in this room bathed in sweat, nervous about being behind with her work and afraid of being exposed as a fraud.

David had suffered a car crash, which was unavoidable. He presented with PTSD. He was asked to relive the car crash in as much detail as possible, and then to review the worst moments, and what they meant to him. He described the appraisals he had made at the moment when the car came to rest after the crash. He had thought "Someone is dead, and it is my fault." The therapist then attempted to help David challenge these ideas, by reviewing the information he had acquired later. In fact no one had been seriously injured, and he was seen by the police as totally blameless. However, he clung to the belief that he had caused it. The therapist inquired about his evidence for this. He explained that he was sure that he had attracted the accident because he was an evil person, and this was a punishment from God. The origin of such appraisals appeared to lie in the experience of his father being mentally ill and repeatedly telling the children that they were bad. One particular episode stuck in his memory: In this his father was screaming at him and saying that he had done something terrible, and God would never forgive him and would find many ways to punish him. He had held this belief for many years and had processed many bad experiences in this light. Thus, to treat his PTSD the therapist had to tackle this set of core beliefs and assumptions. This was done by rescripting his most upsetting childhood memory, as described in Chapter 5. This had a significant effect on his PTSD symptoms that had arisen from the car crash.

When attempting to access key appraisals encapsulated in traumatic memories it has proved rewarding to ask patients to "relive" the memories, evoking them with their eyes closed, and speaking in the first person, present tense. Much more material is elicited than via discussion of the traumatic experience, and the patient may be surprised to recall important details that had previously been forgotten. This useful procedure will be expanded upon in Chapter 5. Following the reliving an inspection of the worst moments or "hot spots" usually reveals important (often distorted) meanings given to events at the time of the trauma, and not updated (Ehlers et al., 2002; Grey et al., 2002).

Michael suffered an unavoidable crash. As the cars came to rest Michael saw the other driver slumped over the wheel. To Michael this meant that he was dead. He felt guilty for months afterwards, tormenting himself with anxiety about whether he might have been able to avert the crash. In fact the driver was shocked but unhurt, and the police had told Michael at the accident scene that the accident was not his fault, and there was no way he could have avoided it.

Thus it appears that (despite the fact that people often have contradictory information at their disposal) when the trauma memories are triggered the *original* appraisals and affect arise. In other cases, close examination of the memories during reliving may reveal images of events that did not in fact occur but were only imagined at the time, or in the light of subsequent upsetting information. Occasionally it transpires that woven into the intrusive memories of a recent trauma is material from a much-earlier trauma, which may have colored meanings given to the recent event.

> Karen (described above) was told by the police that one of her children had lived for an hour after being rescued from the burning building. Karen had an image of him struggling for breath and cried as she described how unfair this seemed, as her son had been born premature and disabled, and had also struggled for breath in the incubator. The therapist decided to ask the firemen about what had happened to the child. They informed her that he had in fact been deeply unconscious immediately after the explosion that caused the fire. Karen's intrusive "memory" of that day (when she was not actually present) owed more to input from an earlier memory than she had realized. However, the image had troubled her deeply for years.

Early memories can play an important part in other Axis I disorders, so reliving is a useful way of exploring the hot cognitions here too. The early memories are first identified by asking the individual about the current felt sense evoked during a recent episode of anxiety, and whether the individual has any memories of past upsetting events that could account for this, or indeed any other memories that are triggered during episodes of anxiety.

Next, the person is asked to relive the distressing childhood memory, in the first person, present tense, and describe everything (including thoughts and emotions) in a lot of detail. Therapist and patient then reflect on the meanings the person gave to this event, and the extent to which the patient still holds these beliefs in the present. Once again the patient may be surprised at the degree of affect and the amount of detail evoked, as in some of the cases described above (see also Hackmann, 2005a; Wild, Hackmann, & Clark, 2007).

Examining the "Felt Sense" When Exposed to Feared Situations

Activating the system so that we can explore meanings while they are "hot" requires the creation of conditions that will trigger them, and the kind of relationship that fosters trust. Our previous discussion would suggest that it is possible to achieve this activation by exposing the person to situational cues. Of course, this is often suggested as homework. However, where practical, accompanying the patient into the real situation provides a great opportunity to catch appraisals "on-line" (see Chapter 6). Again the range of cognitions evoked may surprise the patient and the therapist, encompassing images, body sensations, thoughts, and memories, even in a straightforward problem like a simple phobia.

Once the affect is aroused patients are asked to stay in the situation and tune in to their negative automatic thoughts, images, metaphorical images and thoughts, memories, body state, posture, goals, and plans. Reflection on this material enables meanings to be elicited, concerning the self, the world, and other people.

While doing *in-vivo* exposure, it can be interesting to inquire about bodily sensations and observe gestures and posture. For example, Rosa (described below) refused at first to go anywhere near a spider, or to handle any fruit that might have come from South America. This was because she feared that any spider (particularly one from a foreign country) might contain venom that could kill her. We now describe the work done to examine Rosa's beliefs, highlighting the various aspects of the work that we identified earlier in this chapter.

Rosa had a disabling phobia of spiders, present since she was small. She avoided many situations for fear of encountering spiders. She could not visit friends at home, in case they had dusty houses with cobwebs. If she saw a spider while she was out, she would run away or ask strangers to get rid of it.

She described a *recent, specific episode*, in which she asked someone to get rid of a spider. As it scuttled away, she realized that she was afraid that it now knew where she was, and would go and tell its friends, who would then come and get her. She had a vivid image of this happening and could picture a spider giving her a fatal bite. Next, the therapist provided some *situational cues*, by asking her to attempt to enter a room where a small spider was sitting in a glass jar with a cover over it. Rosa was terrified that the therapist might remove the cover, and the spider would escape and bite her. Even the prospect of seeing the spider was so frightening that she was terrified that she might die of fright. She thought that her heart would jump out of her chest and then she would die.

The therapist made an *emotional bridge* by asking Rosa when in her life she had first had ideas like these. She recounted the experience that triggered her phobia. When she was 4 years old, she was at home with a teenage babysitter, who was watching television. Rosa was playing in the hall, when she heard a noise in the bedroom, although there was no one else in the apartment. Frightened, she ran to the babysitter. Unfortunately, the babysitter happened to be watching the horror film *Arachnophobia*, and was quite scared herself. The two clung together watching terrifying film images of spiders biting people. The imagery Rosa had of spiders suggested input from memory of this early experience.

Armed with this information the therapist and patient were able to do further *behavioral experiments*, to discover whether spiders would behave in the way that Rosa feared, and whether she would die of panic. The therapist visited a zoo with the patient, and they experimented with approaching the display cases with spiders in them, and then handling harmless spiders (with supervision from the keeper). This demonstrated to Rosa that "these spiders don't bite." Her confidence grew as she realized that her fear quickly subsided, and that spiders would not kill her.

It may also be helpful to focus on a patient's posture, and to reflect on its meaning. Patients who were abused or bullied may notice that in trigger situations their posture becomes subservient and they cannot maintain eye contact. The therapy relationship itself, of course, provides a "schema laboratory" within which hot appraisals are likely to be triggered, and can then be examined "on-line."

Judith entered the therapy room and could not meet the therapist's eye. When questioned about this she said that she was scared to look at the therapist because she was afraid there was something different about her, which might mean that she was angry and about to discharge Judith. She was encouraged to describe what she had noticed but could not do so, just saying again that she knew the therapist looked different. When she finally looked at the therapist she realized that all that had changed about her was her hairstyle.

Other Methods of Assessing Meanings

Patients can also be asked to recount or relive dreams and nightmares, with the same purpose of accessing meanings associated with the "hot spots." In PTSD, the themes in nightmares are often closely linked with those in the daytime flashbacks and may incorporate material from other traumatic memories, which are thematically linked. Beck noted similar themes in negative automatic thoughts, daytime imagery, and dreams in depression (Beck & Hurvich, 1959; Beck & Ward, 1961). Research on cognitive themes in dreams has not been done in the anxiety disorders, but clinical experience suggests that similar parallels are observed here, which may be clinically useful.

Sometimes higher order meanings are hard to put into words. One way into the system is via the use of metaphor. Patients may be asked to think about books, pictures, films, and so forth, the themes of which may encapsulate the felt sense they are trying to convey. An imagery technique may also be helpful. The patient is asked to consider an upsetting situation, and bring it to mind. The patient reflects in detail on how this feels emotionally, and what the patient notices is happening in the body. Next, the patient focuses with his or her eyes closed on what a metaphor might be for how he or she feels, and lets a metaphorical image arise. Then the patient considers everything about the image—how it looks; what it looks like close up, or from different angles; its color, texture, and temperature; whether there are any sounds associated with it, or tastes or smells, and so on. The patient is asked to unpack its meaning, reflecting on what (if this is a metaphor for the troublesome situation) this might mean about him or her, other people, and the world. It is also sometimes relevant to explore what the history of this image might be: why this particular image came to mind (Edwards, 1989). All of this work will contribute to the case formulation on which the treatment will be based, and a worksheet is provided in Chapter 5 (where we discuss methods of transforming metaphorical images and their meanings) for therapists interested in accessing and transforming metaphorical images. There are also some interesting metaphors used by patients in the next chapter on formulation.

> A couple came to therapy to address their relationship issues. Each was asked to quietly reflect on how each felt, and provide a metaphor that captured this. James said that his image was of himself rowing the wrong way up the Amazon, with all of his family and their baggage on board, feeling exhausted. Hilda experienced herself as a china doll, elegantly dressed and spinning round for her partner's pleasure, feeling bored and frustrated. These images formed the basis for exploring and adapting their assumptions about their respective roles in the marriage.

CONCLUSION

In straightforward cases it is relatively easy to carry out the kind of detailed assessment that allows one to apply the specific model to the specific case. When idiosyncratic cognitions are present, and when working with atypical or comorbid cases it is important to make an in-depth assessment before making plans about what to target in therapy. This work provides the basis for further collaborative formulation work, as described in Chapter 3.

In this chapter we attempted to formulate the following set of principles for identifying higher order appraisals that need to be targeted in therapy:

- Examine hot material.
- Notice what triggered the upsetting feelings.
- Consider specific examples. This will achieve more than general discussion.
- Explore the whole felt sense: images, memories, body sensations, posture, gesture, metaphor, and so on.
- In some cases it may be interesting and useful to make a bridge to the past, and see how input from memory is coloring the present.
- Intrusive memories and memories discovered to be providing input to current intrusive imagery can be relived, to access hot spots and their meanings.
- Dreams, nightmares, and the use of metaphor can also be informative and the therapeutic relationship can provide a "schema laboratory."
- Metacognitive appraisals of contents of consciousness and associated covert and overt safety behaviors should be examined.
- Special note should be taken of broad themes arising in therapy, as these will prove useful in deriving a formulation.

THREE

Case Formulation
Making Sense of Complexity

A case formulation, or conceptualization, is a way to make sense of a particular patient's problems. Making a formulation is not "fitting someone to a formula" but using one's knowledge of the theory and employing a wide array of clinical sensitivities and skills to develop a hypothesis, together with the patient, about how a problem developed, how episodes of difficulty are triggered, and how the problem is maintained. In old-fashioned terms, it should address predisposing, precipitating, and perpetuating factors and guide decisions about treatment. The words "formulation" and "conceptualization" are often used interchangeably. The word "formulation" is the one that is used here.

This chapter focuses on the difficulty of producing clear, theoretically sound, and useful formulations when working with atypical or complex cases. These are cases in which there is a high incidence of comorbidity, for example, between different manifestations of anxiety, between anxiety and depression, or between anxiety and one or more of the personality disorders. Such complexity makes it hard to understand and to make sense of presenting problems in terms of the theoretical links between all the relevant factors. Sometimes information may be lacking; often problems appear not to hang together, and it is not usually possible to apply theory to the case in the relatively straightforward way illustrated so well by the specific cognitive-behavioral models for single, specific, anxiety disorders that we outlined in Chapter 1.

In less straightforward and also in unusual cases there is a risk that therapists will construct increasingly complex formulations, and that the end product will then lose some of its potential clinical value. The more complex a formulation, the harder it is for the patient and the therapist to understand, to remember, and to use as a basis for making theoretically sound decisions about what action is likely to help. The two main solutions to this problem suggested in this chapter are closely linked: to keep the formulation as simple as possible and to learn to think about deeper levels of patient cognition, about beliefs as well as about thoughts and assumptions. As we saw in Chapter 2, a thorough assessment is needed so as to understand cognitive factors in depth. In this chapter we present strategies and tools for helping clinicians to use the products of this assessment in their formulation work.

PRINCIPLES GUIDING CASE FORMULATION

Three central principles guide the case formulation process (for further discussion see Butler, 1998, 1999a; Johnstone, 2006). A clear understanding of these principles, and of their implications, is essential when working with complex cases.

1. A formulation should be *based on a theory*, reflecting an attempt to put the theory into practice. Working this way enhances consistency, allows therapists to draw on the same basic theory irrespective of the specific emotion they are working with (such as anxiety or depression, or mixtures of anxiety anger and shame), and helps them when stuck to think about what the theory would suggest: for example, that this person often feels threatened and vulnerable even though it is as yet difficult to define triggers of specific episodes of anxiety or links between presenting problems.

2. A formulation should be *hypothetical* in nature, so that it can be modified by information gained during the course of treatment—and also so that patients can be invited to contribute, asked for their feedback, and encouraged to collaborate in searching for a way of making sense. (Therapists should avoid making pronouncements: "this is how it is," etc.). This also recognizes that there may be more than one possibility, and that the interaction between diverse factors, such as genetic predisposition, cultural pressures, and reactions to frightening experiences, may be hard to disentangle.

3. A formulation should be as *parsimonious* as possible—for the sake of simplicity, clarity, and ease of remembering. The more complex the formulation, and the representation of it, the harder it will be to remember, and the harder it will be to use (for the patient as well as for the therapist). This is one of the central points made in this chapter and it is discussed further below (pp. 62–64).

APPLYING THESE PRINCIPLES TO RESOLVE PROBLEMS IN FORMULATION

When applying these principles to resolve problems in formulation it is essential to be able to draw on the generic cognitive model (Beck, 1976). As cognitive therapists we understand a wide range of problems, including anxiety, in terms of general theories about the links between cognition, behavior, physiology, and affect. A standard way of representing this model for the purposes of formulation is shown next. This is represented diagrammatically in the top half of Figure 3.1, and in the bottom half this general model is applied to a patient with complex GAD.

This way of making sense of a particular patient's concerns continues to have value when working with complex and treatment-resistant cases. There are, however, two other ways of making sense: through diagnosis and through using one of the more specific models described in Chapter 1. These different ways of making sense serve different functions and have different advantages and disadvantages (Butler, 1998). In straightforward cases all three fit well together: A diagnosis of social phobia defines

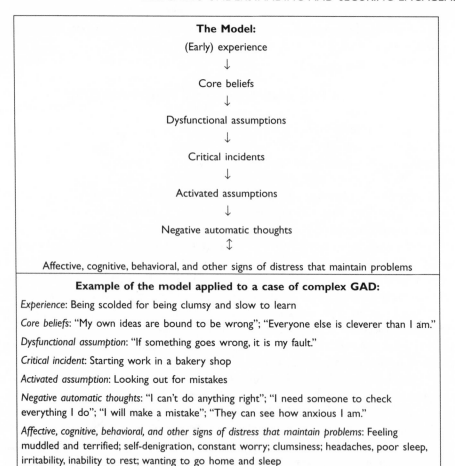

The Model:

(Early) experience

↓

Core beliefs

↓

Dysfunctional assumptions

↓

Critical incidents

↓

Activated assumptions

↓

Negative automatic thoughts

↕

Affective, cognitive, behavioral, and other signs of distress that maintain problems

Example of the model applied to a case of complex GAD:

Experience: Being scolded for being clumsy and slow to learn

Core beliefs: "My own ideas are bound to be wrong"; "Everyone else is cleverer than I am."

Dysfunctional assumption: "If something goes wrong, it is my fault."

Critical incident: Starting work in a bakery shop

Activated assumption: Looking out for mistakes

Negative automatic thoughts: "I can't do anything right"; "I need someone to check everything I do"; "I will make a mistake"; "They can see how anxious I am."

Affective, cognitive, behavioral, and other signs of distress that maintain problems: Feeling muddled and terrified; self-denigration, constant worry; clumsiness; headaches, poor sleep, irritability, inability to rest; wanting to go home and sleep

FIGURE 3.1. The cognitive model and its application to a case of complex GAD.

features of the presenting problem; application of the Clark and Wells (1995) model suggests how these fit together and indicates which processes (e.g., self-focused attention, safety behaviors) serve important maintaining functions; and the formulation specifies how the social anxiety is manifested and maintained in the particular case (e.g., through attempting to monitor signs of trembling and shaking, and through speaking quietly in an attempt not to attract attention).

In this book we are considering how to proceed when complexities interfere with the straightforward application of such clearly specified procedures, and this tends to happen when the various ways of making sense no longer fit together so smoothly. For example, more than one diagnosis may apply, or there may be no single diagnosis that fits the particular case; there may be no specific model for the problems presented by the patient, or the anxiety problems may be just one aspect of a complex set of problems following early childhood trauma, and so on. Here the case formulation is the main—or even the only—source of ideas about how, in theory, to understand presenting problems, and how to provide an effective treatment. This gives case formulations, and the work that goes into developing them, a central role in determining the process of therapy as well as the content (see also Tarrier, 2006).

Even in straightforward cases, making a formulation involves using clinical judgment. In unusual, complex, and comorbid cases, or when information is missing, therapists are increasingly dependent on their clinical judgment. Safeguards are therefore needed to ensure that mistaken ideas are not being imposed on patients. The work needs to be done together—in collaboration, and the style of cognitive therapy plays a crucial role here. Being explicit about how we understand what we have been told provides one kind of check, provided that we have also taken care to ensure that our patients are able to give us honest and detailed feedback. For example, some patients have a strong "need to please." Others are fearful of offending their therapists and keep their doubts to themselves. Then it is especially important to adopt the Socratic style of questioning, and to use methods to guide discovery. It is important to give people enough time to consider, and to ask questions that help them become genuinely engaged in constructing a (theoretically consistent) way of making sense of their difficulties. We need to find out at each stage, for instance, whether the current formulation seems coherent to them, and whether they can draw on it as a source of ideas about how to change. Some examples of useful questions to assist in making the process of formulation a collaborative enterprise are shown in Figure 3.2.

Patients are the most obvious source of comment on our developing case formulations. Other sounding boards include supervisors and colleagues, and a degree of objectivity can also be found by using behavioral experiments to test specific hypotheses relevant to a formulation (Bennett-Levy, Butler, et al., 2004; Wells, 1997). We discuss the use of behavioral experiments at length in Chapter 6. In addition, there may be results from new research or theoretical developments to take into account, such as Borkovec's (2007) findings concerning the value of attending to interpersonal and experiential processes during treatment for GAD.

Making links:
  "How does that fit together? Could that link up with . . . ?"

Looking for patterns and themes:
  "Is there a pattern here? Is that a pattern?"

Exploring meanings:
  "How do you make sense of that? How do you understand it?"
  "What are the implications of that for you?"
  "What does that mean to you?"
  "What kind of impact does / did that have on you?"

Clarifying processes and mechanisms:
  "What do you think keeps this going?"
  "And when that happens, what do you think / feel / do / conclude?"
  "When you do that, how do you feel? At the time? Later on?"
  "If you think . . . , what do you then do?"

FIGURE 3.2. Examples of formulation-based questions.

ANXIETY DISORDERS AND FORMULATION WORK:
MAPPING THE TERRITORY

There is a basic tension in working to formulate particular cases, as it involves bridging the gap between relatively simple, clear theoretical models and the largely unknown, complex, and private world of the person who is anxious. The first essential step is paying close attention to each person's experience of anxiety, and tuning in to that person's particular sense of feeling at risk, under threat, or in danger. To apply the principles concerning the use of theory, hypotheses, and parsimony to resolve problems in formulation it also helps to broaden our understanding of anxiety, and to share that understanding with our patients. Many people can tell us why they become anxious, but there are also many who cannot do so. They may be confused by their experiences and unable to predict when their symptoms will occur. The task of case formulation is harder in such cases and can be helped by drawing on information about anxiety beyond that represented in each of the specific models. Four general points about anxiety that have important implications for the task of formulation are described next.

Anxiety Has Secondary Consequences

Anxiety has secondary consequences, especially if it has been present for a long time. These include depression, impaired confidence, and reduced self-esteem. Making the distinction between primary and secondary features of presenting problems helps to reduce confusion. It also helps make sense of the secondary features and clarifies how to target interventions. It is, after all, not surprising that persistent anxiety "gets people down," undermines their confidence in their own abilities, and reduces their sense of self-worth. The cognitive model of low self-esteem, which takes particular account of comorbid anxiety and depression, can sometimes be helpful here (see Chapter 8).

Different Manifestations of Anxiety Are Often Linked

There are conceptual links among the different kinds of anxiety in the DSM, despite the distinctions. For example, whatever problems your anxiety brings, you can *worry* about them. Worry tends to spread from one thing to another, and aspects of GAD are often present even in the absence of the full clinical version of the problem. Similarly, people are often embarrassed by their anxiety problems and feel *at risk of being judged or rejected by others* because of them. This adds a social dimension to their anxiety. So we need a way of formulating that helps to make sense of the whole picture, including attitudes and reactions to anxiety, rather than just part of it. This should include consideration of a person's relative strengths and assets, as recognizing these early on helps to reverse the effects of low self-confidence and low self-esteem, validates and affirms the person so as to increase motivation, and increases awareness of skills to draw on during treatment. It provides a general, confidence-building framework for treatment based on efforts to construct (or strengthen) adaptive functioning, which is not focused exclusively on reducing (or demolishing) unhelpful thoughts and behaviors.

Some of the accepted wisdom about which problems should be tackled first may be exactly that: (accepted) assumptions rather than the product of research. Common assumptions are that depression should be treated before anxiety, social anxiety before worry, alcohol misuse before anxiety, and panic (or Axis I disorders generally) before personality disorder (and Axis II disorders generally). Yet in our research on the treatment of GAD we found that treating the GAD also reduced depression scores (from an average BDI [Beck Depression Inventory] score of 21.4 to an average of 7.5 after treatment; Butler, Fennell, Robson, & Gelder, 1991), and clinical observations during this research trial indicated that changes in depression rapidly followed engagement in treatment, possibly reflecting increased hope that the main problem could be alleviated. One possible explanation is that broad understanding of anxiety and of the ways in which problems interrelate, together with skilled case-formulation work that takes assets as well as deficits into account, facilitates change across as well as within problems. What we have come to think of as separate and distinct may not be so separate in practice, and these assumptions can be tested clinically as well as in research.

Earlier Experiences May Explain Specific Triggers of Anxiety

Particular events such as turning aside or snapping a finger may trigger anxiety because of their links with earlier experiences. For example, one patient, Rachel, became anxious if the person she was talking to looked away. This small action triggered an intense fear of being left unacknowledged and abandoned because of her childhood experiences.

Formulating such idiosyncratic meanings is essential and difficult and often involves paying close attention to events within the therapeutic relationship. Small behavior changes can provoke disproportionate reactions, and these small behavioral events often take some time to notice during therapy, and which can be difficult to make sense of. It can be relatively easy to feel and to notice the disruption to the therapy process (Rachel's silence when she felt abandoned), but harder to understand its cause (the therapist looking away). The patient may not find it easy, for many reasons, to explain the process as it affects them, and clinical judgment is needed to decide how and when to explore these observations in order jointly to ascertain their significance. Such explorations will also be more difficult when experiences are stored in implicit memory and are hard to put into words. Then it can be especially useful to use drawings, metaphor, or imagery to represent the "felt sense" (see Chapter 2 for a detailed discussion of this issue).

Three Common Reactions to Anxiety: Control, Rigidity, and Safety-Seeking

Our understanding of anxiety in broad terms suggests there are three common reactions to feeling anxious: a wish to keep control, a tendency to rigidity in responsiveness, and the desire to seek safety or protection. As therapists, our starting point is that anxiety is about feeling threatened or at risk. The danger has not yet occurred, but it could, so there is necessarily a degree of uncertainty about what might happen and/or about how one might cope with it, whether the threat or risk is internal or external (see also Chapter 9). An understandable reaction to this uncertainty is to try to keep control.

There is also a well-documented tendency for people to become increasingly rigid or inflexible in their reactions when anxious (see, e.g., Borkovec & Newman, 1998). A reduced range of responsiveness has been found in autonomic, behavioral and cognitive responses, and also in measures of electroencephalogram (EEG) activity (specifically for people who suffer from GAD—but we have already noted the pervasiveness of worry). The messages that we give our children in many Western cultures as they grow up and encounter alarming situations may also encourage them to "hang in there," "keep going," "batten down the hatches," and generally to persist in the face of fear (to "get a grip," and maintain a stiff upper lip). These messages may encourage the development of tension and rigidity as responses to anxiety, as if that could assist in getting a handle on the fear and prevent it surging out of control. Finally, seeking safety or protection leads to familiar patterns of avoidance, to safety behaviors, to escape behaviors and thoughts about escape, and sometimes even to dissociation.

Formulation work should therefore start by recognizing that these general reactions make sense. The task is to explore idiosyncratic versions of them in a particular case, and to consider how best to replace them with more functional reactions. Three general aims or themes may guide this work, and help to determine new attitudes to the understanding and treatment of anxiety. These are to encourage curiosity rather than control, to increase flexibility and reduce rigidity, and to learn how to face (and accept) fears and anxiety, rather than seeking (too much) safety and protection. These aims provide a broad context within which to apply the strategies derived from specific models.

The four aspects of anxiety described above provide a way of thinking in terms of commonalities across specific anxiety disorders. In addition, therapists can draw on general psychological principles. For example, we know that novelty triggers anxiety, in humans and animals: As familiarity develops it becomes easier to explore, signs of anxiety diminish, and signs of feeling safe and confident increase. From the point of view of someone with a personality disorder, or with a history of repeatedly being subjected to dangerous or threatening situations, intense anxiety may occur if familiar patterns change, even if the novelty is potentially positive. People may be fearful of abstractions or generalities, such as the sense that things feel unpredictable or out of control, or they may feel anxious if they do not know what to expect, or what to do, or what others expect of them and so on.

It follows that intense anxiety may erupt if something familiar changes, or threatens to change, and that it will be important to help such people to develop a sense of security (or of "safeness" in Gilbert's [2005a, p. 22] terminology) before or, as well as, encouraging them to confront their fears directly. The arguments above also suggest that a person presenting with comorbidity, when anxiety coexists with affective or with personality disorders, will be more efficiently treated when their problems are formulated in terms of core beliefs that are common to the different presenting problems. Work on changing these beliefs would then, theoretically, be likely to result in a variety of different changes simultaneously. As one patient with numerous anxiety problems, low self-esteem, and a history of abusive relationships put it: "It's like moving on all fronts at once."

JUDGING THE QUALITY OF A CASE FORMULATION

If formulation work is to play a central role in solving problems that arise when treating anxiety, then clearly our formulations should be good ones, and we should double-check the information on which they are based and reformulate when we fail to get the desired or expected results. However, judging the quality of a case formulation is a complex business. An incomplete formulation can still be useful. So can one that is wrong, for example, when it assists in narrowing down the possibilities, or when it prompts patients to clarify misunderstanding and enhances their ability to give honest feedback, or when talking about it prompts recollection of previously undisclosed material. For these reasons case formulations should be judged not only in terms of the qualities of the finished product (internal consistency, accuracy with respect to the facts, predictive power, etc.) but also with respect to the dynamic processes involved in making and using them, and taking account of the success with which helpful metamessages are delivered, for example, about the factors contributing to the development of problems. When reflecting on a piece of formulation work one might consider, for example, whether it engaged a process of exploration, increased pattern-recognition skills, brought order out of confusion, revealed new options, secured a feeling of being understood, and helped to clarify and predict process issues and future problems. The work of developing a formulation is thus different from and potentially more valuable than the end product (the final version), which may be written down and evaluated, but may also live only in the therapists' head, or notes.

Current research on the interrater reliability of case formulations has not yet produced clear-cut results (e.g., Bieling & Kuyken, 2003; Eells, Kendjelic, & Lucas, 1998; Fothergill & Kuyken, 2003; Persons & Bertagnolli, 1999; Persons, Mooney, & Padesky, 1995). This is not surprising given the complex processes involved. If we are to be able to justify our clinical decisions and be held accountable for them, we still need to use our theories, and specific models when they are available, to make sense of the information presented to us. So even if our belief in the value of case formulations and of formulation work, generally, is largely a matter of faith, it remains important that therapists reliably make and use them. Faced with someone's continued anxiety despite one's best efforts to help, we can then reformulate and check that our actions and interventions are based on (theoretically based) hypotheses rather than on hunches and habits. This is especially important when a therapist and a patient make sense of things in different ways. Explicitly phrasing the different views as hypotheses to explore then provides the basis, for example, for further information gathering and experiment. A patient with multiple anxieties following a disrupted and unstable childhood commented: "At first making sense was not a lot of help. Once I started to change I could see it was the key." The process of case formulation is thus essentially dynamic, and the interactive and changing processes involved will have to be taken into account before we can find out more about the value of the work that goes into making sense of someone's difficulties. "Formulation work" may be as important as, or more important than, the end product.

An example of a patient's reflections on the value of formulation work is to be found in P. S. (2006, and discussed in Butler, 2006). The patient told us that "Formulation is a tool that was used in my treatment. I found it enormously helpful. At the beginning I had a mixture of rational and irrational beliefs and assumptions. I could not discriminate between them. They all had equal internal authority in determining my actions. The formulation made the incomprehensible accessible. It explained and imparted insight. I understood myself" (p. 13).

USING METAPHORS, PICTURES, AND DIAGRAMS
IN FORMULATION WORK

In atypical cases formulation work is likely to be harder, and its dynamic aspects are especially important. There are also different ways of proceeding with formulation work, and different ways may suit different circumstances. So therapists faced with complicated or unusual manifestations of anxiety need to be flexible in their approach to making and using formulations. Sometimes it is useful to emphasize systemic factors and ideas about patterns of relating to and interacting with other people; at others it may help to start from a problem list, or it may be more helpful to be selective, and to focus solely on the main problems. Often therapists initially base their formulations on a maintaining cycle in the present and work backwards from there, including assumptions and beliefs as required. But sometimes it might be better (or easiest) to gather an overall impression of a patient's particular perspective, and to begin by making a hypothesis about underlying beliefs: This person had a terrible life story and learned early on never to trust people. Therefore therapy needs to start by building trust, and looking at patient behaviors in the present. For example, being unwilling to disclose personal information or defensive can (tentatively) be fitted into the case formulation as making sense in terms of underlying cognitive structures. The cognitive processes involved, for example in mistrust, might also be expected to interfere with the process of gathering the detailed information needed for formulation work based more exclusively on less abstract cognitive processes. This is not to say that other things might not also be going on, nor is it to say that this hypothesis is right, but it provides a (collaborative) starting point, and that is what it is meant to do. We have no information yet to suggest that one starting point is better than another.

Pictures, stories, metaphors, and diagrams can all help in the task of formulating and contribute to making sense, and often our patients provide us with useful tools in the metaphors and images they bring to treatment. A deeply avoidant patient who dreaded talking or thinking about her fears and her current situation described herself as hidden in a huge bramble bush. She felt as if she was surrounded by a thicket that had grown up around her so tightly that she did not dare to open her eyes for fear of the thorns. This made some sense in terms of the dangerous situation that she had endured as a child, and her fear of discovering just how painful it would be to extract herself. However her situation was now different, and her combined safety behaviors and avoidance were preventing her noticing the difference: Metaphorically speaking she could not open her eyes and look around. The metaphor was further elaborated without losing touch with the underlying theory.

Another patient found it hard to understand how, during a setback in her progress, all her old problems reemerged, one by one, until she "ground to a halt." She made sense of this by saying it was like being on an old-fashioned train. When it stopped all the separate carriages bumped one at a time into those in front, giving the passengers a series of jolts. She decided she would no longer be a passenger but restart the train and keep it moving. The metaphor revealed her current perspective, assisted in the reevaluation of this, and helped her to adopt a different attitude that then provided a basis for specific behavioral changes.

These metaphors are listed first to emphasize the point that there is no single way of formulating more complex cases, and no precise model available to ease the therapist's task. Further illustrations are provided in the next two chapters. For some people relatively standard methods may work well (e.g., Butler, 1998; Eells, 1997, 2006; Nezu, Nezu, & Lombardo, 2004; Persons, 1989; Westbrook, Kennerley, & Kirk, 2007). Here we have selected a few of the many possible diagrammatic representations of elements of formulation work and we present them as illustrations of useful tools rather than templates (Figures 3.3–3.8).

The diagram in Figure 3.3 represents a way of formulating a habitual process of interaction between people that reveals its self-defeating effect. This pattern has clear implications for what to do: learn to recognize the pattern, change the old behavior (in this case, being nice to everybody), and find out what happens. It also reveals a common difficulty: When people try to change such patterns they sometimes go to extremes and need to learn more appropriate and flexible ways of behaving that fall in the middle ground between being nice to everyone and saying what you think however offensive that might be.

In Figure 3.4 there is a visual representation of patterns of cognition similar to those described by Padesky (1993a) in her article about self-prejudice. The "Mental Crusher" stands at the entrance to the schematic head and allows information consistent with prevailing ideas readily to be processed and stored (rectangular shapes). It operates so as to force inconsistent information (the other shapes) into the same shape. If the information remains a different shape it will be ignored or forgotten. Only information that naturally fits, or has been distorted to fit, can enter. The whole picture can be used to explain why nothing changes. In practice this will need to be illustrated, amplified, and tested using specific examples. One patient spoke, for instance, about numerous comments and requests made by her boss, reporting them as evidence for his critical view of her work and her abilities. With the Mental Crusher in mind she agreed to pay more careful attention to his actual words. It soon became clear that she had been ignoring appreciative or encouraging remarks, assuming that he was only being nice to her. In her view, he did not really mean them so they meant nothing to her. At the same time his neutral remarks or behaviors, such as accepting her work without comment or ignoring her while she got on with the work, were interpreted by her as criticisms—distorted to fit.

Figure 3.5 provides a schematic representation of the way in which someone's early experience may have led to a particular way of behaving that elicits the kinds of reactions from others that maintain the behavior. For example, someone whose parents always doubted his competence and scolded him for making mistakes developed a habit of apologizing repeatedly, even when nothing had gone wrong. When his therapist noticed this he started counting and calculated that early in treatment the patient

"I want to be liked."
↓
"I must be nice to everybody."
↓
"I can't be myself."
↓
"I can never know if people like me."

FIGURE 3.3. A self-defeating pattern of interaction.

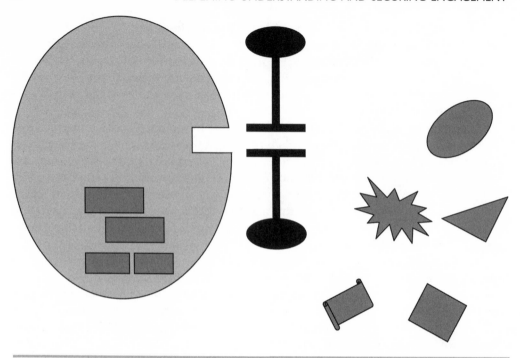

FIGURE 3.4. The Mental Crusher.

said "sorry" 37 times in just under 30 minutes. The diagram suggests that this behavior elicits reactions from others that maintain it: The more he apologized, the more others doubted his competence. The more they doubted him, the more he apologized. When asked if this made sense, this patient provided a specific example. He had borrowed his neighbor's lawn mower and returned it in good order. A couple of weeks later the mower broke down when the neighbor was using it. The patient (feeling highly anxious) apologized and was accused of having caused the problem. When asked to pay for repairs, he avoided discussion and paid up, assuming he must be responsible (even though he could not think how).

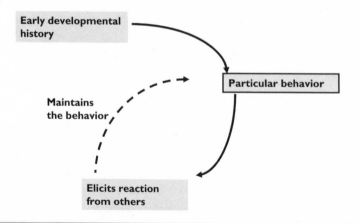

FIGURE 3.5. Schematic representation of a historical process.

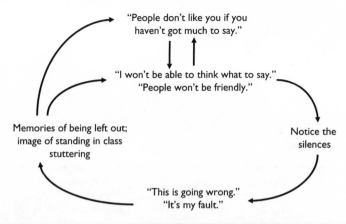

"People don't like you if you
haven't got much to say."

"I won't be able to think what to say."
"People won't be friendly."

Memories of being left out;
image of standing in class
stuttering

Notice the
silences

"This is going wrong."
"It's my fault."

FIGURE 3.6. How to collect a store of information that fits with what you already know.

Figure 3.6 illustrates another way of representing cognitive maintaining processes, based on that described by Fennell (1999, p. 43; see also Chapter 4, p. 80). This draws attention to the ways in which assumptions, perceptions, interpretations, and memory interact. These parsimonious representations of complex interactions can clarify maintaining processes. Further work may be needed to identify relevant thoughts and feelings, but even before this has been done, outline sketches such as these may be sufficient to engage someone in the process of trying out new ways of behaving. The information this provides can then contribute to more detailed formulation work.

The diagram in Figure 3.7 also makes use of the principle of parsimony and illustrates in outline how many different kinds of processes may be generated by an underlying belief and contribute to its maintenance. Last, Figure 3.8 illustrates the value of selecting two levels of cognition so as to illustrate their differences and their interrelatedness. In the example, one of these represents a schema, and the other represents the ways in which this person attempts to prevent the schema being activated. This sketch can also be used to illustrate how the different levels of cognition are associated with different kinds of affect. In the example provided, activating the schema evoked intense sadness. Efforts to prevent the schema being activated were motivated by anxiety. Recognizing these links helped to explain why attempts to change such behaviors felt so alarming.

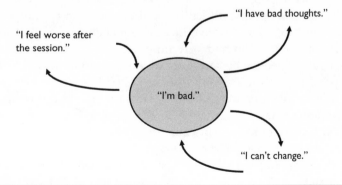

"I have bad thoughts."

"I feel worse after
the session."

"I'm bad."

"I can't change."

FIGURE 3.7. Making sense of similar processes.

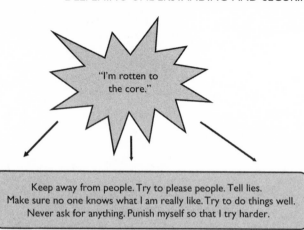

FIGURE 3.8. Illustrating links between two levels of cognition.

Of course verbal descriptions as well as metaphors and diagrams can help in the infinitely various process of making sense. Someone with "borderline features" to her problems, who suffered intensely from anxiety, described having the feeling that she was her own worst enemy, as whenever she started to improve she did something to make things worse again. Unpacking this process of "self-sabotage" provided her with a new hypothesis: making functional changes in her life (providing an organizational framework and structure to her day) put her in unfamiliar territory, which felt strange and alarming. The more novel her situation, the less safe and the more scared she felt. Reestablishing old (familiar) behaviors such as drinking too much alcohol and cutting her legs made her feel safe again. Further work was needed on learning how to comfort herself, and on establishing more functional and enduring ways of providing a sense that she could be safe and secure in this world. Understanding the processes involved also helped her to accept and to tolerate a degree of anxiety, and to accept a slower rate of change.

FORMULATING INTERACTIONS BETWEEN PEOPLE

The principles of formulation work described and illustrated so far apply just as well to the interactions between people as to the individual case. They can help us to understand and make sense of specific difficulties and problems in relationships (including the therapy relationship), and to derive ideas about change from that understanding.

For example, a patient who had very little sense of her own value or worth had found that she could cope well by caring for others instead of herself, and by avoiding discussion of painful issues, especially if these linked to her experience of emotional neglect and criticism during childhood. She became highly anxious in interpersonal situations. Her therapist readily recognized her distress and was concerned to set her at ease during their first encounters. Subsequently she found herself making extra efforts to care for and help this patient, and she hesitated to bring up painful material for discussion. Indeed she apologized to the patient when a behavioral experiment elicited much higher anxiety than expected, and the patient responded with caring and concerned remarks about the therapist.

Supervision and self-reflection (Bennett-Levy & Thwaites, 2007) can help to clarify and to formulate such processes. In this case the therapist and the patient were caught up in parallel needs to care for others that reinforced their joint avoidance of topics that might elicit distress. The pattern was discussed explicitly, using material from a recent therapy session. Recognising the "pull" (see, e.g., Safran & Segal, 1990, p. 74) and resisting it during subsequent sessions enabled the therapist to provide a different interpersonal context within which the patient was able to address the issues that she found distressing, and learn to care better for herself.

FORMULATING COMORBIDITY
WITH DIFFERENT KINDS OF ANXIETY

Sometimes it is hard to work out how to apply the principles derived from research, and sometimes doing so fails to bring about the desired—or expected—degree of change. How then should we proceed when a patient has a collection of anxiety symptoms that span specific disorders such as panic attacks, fears of social interactions, and worry? An option discussed by Barlow, Craske, Rapee, and others in a symposium on the topic (Craske, Farchione, Tsao, & Mystkowski, 1998) is to target the anxiety problems successively. For example, to start by focusing on the "main" problem, assessing the degree of change across all relevant anxiety disorders immediately after treatment and after a follow-up interval, and then to target remaining anxiety problems separately, as required. The successive approach illustrates well the influence of thinking predominantly in terms of differentiating features of anxiety states. Similarly, Williams, Watts, MacLeod, and Mathews (1997) explored differentiating features of anxiety and depression that are also often dealt with separately, in research and in the clinic. However, to solve the problem of comorbidity efficiently we may need to think more in terms of commonalities (Hertel, 2002, 2004; Mineka, Walsh, & Clark, 1988; Mogg & Bradley, 1998, 2004).

Formulations have many levels, summarized by Persons (1989) as "overt difficulties" and "underlying mechanisms." The cognitions involved in these underlying mechanisms are usually represented in a hierarchy by cognitive therapists. At the lowest hierarchical level are the many automatic thoughts, positive, negative, and neutral, that represent the "stream of consciousness." Higher up come assumptions; above them beliefs, and finally representations of schemas (variously described). An obvious point follows: Changing cognitions at a higher level in the pyramid will affect a broader range of cognitions lower down. So, in cases of comorbidity, working at higher levels of cognition should enable therapists to target related problems simultaneously rather than successively. An example follows.

Paula, age 28, is in a rocky relationship. She is underconfident at work, and her first presenting problem is that she is unable to go into town, or travel beyond her immediate neighborhood on her own. She has panic attacks at home and also when she is out, and manages to work and to cope at home only with considerable support from her mother and partner. It soon becomes clear that there is also a social aspect to Paula's anxiety: She "knows that others judge and evaluate her"—negatively of course—and is fearful of talking to her boss, of interacting with colleagues, and of socializing in general. In addition, Paula is a worrier. She can worry about anything and everything (e.g., what to buy from the supermarket, arrangements for meeting up with a friend, tidying up, possible future financial difficulties, etc.). On one occasion, following a minor infection, the worry focused on her stomach, and she interpreted each twinge or grumble as a sign of serious illness. She repeatedly sought reassurance, which irritated her partner and provoked arguments, and further worries about the stability and suitability of her relationship.

Paula suffers from numerous forms of anxiety. The therapist started by focusing on Paula's sense of vulnerability and working to understand (formulate) the idiosyncratic flavor of this vulnerability. To begin with, Paula described this by saying, "I can never be confident," a phrase that suggests some underlying beliefs and assumptions. The therapist helped Paula identify these attitudes and assumptions about how or whether confidence develops. This was done partly through Socratic questioning, asking Paula to think about how she had become confident about her ability to type and to drive. It was also done independently by Paula through homework assignments involving discussions with others and behavioral experiments. Her conclusions following this work were that "confidence is not all of a piece." She meant that you can be confident in one area of life but not in another, that confidence can develop and fluctuate, and that many people appear more confident than they feel. Clearly her therapist could have explained this to her straight away, but it is unlikely that this would have had the emotional impact provided by guided discovery and personal experience. Paula started to improve slowly and later observed that as her beliefs about confidence changed, her panic, her social fears, and her worrying all started to decrease. First she opened her mind to the possibility that she might after all be able to achieve a degree of confidence, then the different aspects of her anxiety started to change together. The treatment strategy derived from using a more general, or higher level formulation. It was designed to ensure that all subsequent work was relevant to changing underlying beliefs whatever the associated feelings, specific triggering incidents, or focus for homework between sessions.

Notice that a case formulation does not have to be complete to be useful. One of Paula's early homework tasks was to ask herself, whenever she felt "bad" (anxious, irritable, miserable, etc.): "How does this fit with not being confident?" At this stage she was testing the relevance to her of one (tentative) way of phrasing her underlying sense of vulnerability. Without the incomplete formulation she would not have had this task to perform, and without this task she would have been much less actively involved in the process of case formulation, and more of a passive recipient of someone else's (possibly mistaken) ideas. She might also have focused "down" onto the specifics of each triggering situation, running the risk of becoming overwhelmed by detail, and thus narrowing the possibilities for generalization.

The Skills of Abstraction and Selection

The value of working on underlying (or higher order) meanings cannot be overemphasized. So therapists need to develop skills for thinking at higher levels of abstraction. As Teasdale (1997) said: "You can't change things by thinking at a single level of cognitive architecture," and "We need to become poets in therapy, as the business is about changing higher level, implicational meanings [and] to do this we can use parables, stories and metaphors." The proliferation of multilevel theoretical approaches (e.g., Brewin et al., 1996; Power & Dalgleish, 1997; Teasdale & Barnard, 1993) now provides ways of thinking coherently about the different levels. All of which can contribute to our formulation work—but only if it is seen as a source of (testable) hypotheses rather than as an objectively valid road map. As the example of Paula illustrates, higher level formulation in terms of beliefs about confidence simplified and focused work that might otherwise have become fragmented or overcomplicated.

Consistent with the hierarchical understanding of cognitions generally we would assume that numerous automatic thoughts are influenced by fewer assumptions, which in turn are influenced by fewer beliefs. When formulations provide ideas about higher level, implicational meanings, they will be more likely to assist therapist and patient to achieve lasting change (see also Chapters 2 and 5).

The process of formulation also requires therapists to develop the skill of being able to select from the information available to them. Selection affects every aspect of therapy. Patients select what to focus on, what to talk about in therapy, and what not to disclose. Therapists select what to attend to, what to inquire about, and what to ignore. The therapist's theoretical understanding provides a rationale for further selection. So if the problem is understood as being primarily one of social anxiety, associated depression, irritation, or low self-esteem might (at first) be ignored. So when the focus is on removing maintaining factors, therapists need to focus on a few target cognitions and behaviors and not diffuse the effort by employing a wide spectrum of techniques directed to a range of target behaviors. Recognizing this process of selectivity, and the need for targeting interventions efficiently when anxiety does not resolve, it is useful to think again about how the various kinds of selectivity may have influenced the current formulation and the subsequent choice of treatment methods.

> More often than not, our clients recognize that things are not working in their life but are either unclear as to why or have developed explanations that are erroneous. Metaphorically speaking, they are in the dark about relevant aspects of their functioning (e.g., their emotional reactions) and the functioning of others (e.g., how their emotional reactions impact on others). Our role is to focus a spotlight on those aspects about which we, as their therapists, believe that a better or more accurate awareness would be helpful. Still another way to look at this is that we function as "attention deployers," in that we help clients to become more aware of those thoughts, actions and desires that are relevant to the problems they are experiencing. (Goldfried, 2004, p. 98)

Clearly theoretical considerations should guide the deployment of that clinical spotlight. However, when focusing it we are often more in the dark than we should like to be; theories do not tell us all we would like to know, yet. Detailed supporting evidence may not be available. Patients may communicate in obscure, allusive, or incomplete ways. Information gathered from the processes that operate between patient and therapist may be crucial (and, e.g., reveal problems with dependency or mistrust that help to make sense of the anxiety), but they may also confound the contributions of patient and therapist. If they are to use the processes of selectivity well, therapists as well as their patients need enhanced reflective and metacognitive abilities. They need to use these abilities to reflect on the processes of selection, and on the various biases and heuristics that may be involved in the process of selection.

The Sandwich Principle: A General Formulation Strategy

A sandwich provides a useful metaphor for a general formulation strategy that can help "when the protocols fail." The idea is that a formulation, just like a sandwich, will hold together better, and serve its intended function better, if it has two slices of bread to hold it together. With two slices of bread in place the sandwich can be infinitely various: any shape or size, with any of a myriad different types of filling and so on. Without the two slices of bread the sandwich will fall apart. In the case of the formulation, one slice of bread stands for "beliefs," and the other stands for "behaviors." With beliefs and behavior in mind, it matters less if the focus of therapy shifts between sessions, and the maximum possible change can be elicited even from small behavioral experiments. The following examples are intended to illustrate more clearly what is meant by this metaphor. One general point is that all formulations should include hypotheses about underlying beliefs and ideas about how behaviors can maintain problems. (These provide the basis for further hypotheses about how changing beliefs could help to resolve the problems.) The sandwich principle can be used to hold treatment together if, whenever focusing on a behavior the therapist asks: "How does this fit with your belief that . . . ?" And conversely, whenever focusing on a belief the therapist asks: "How does this link with what you do; with your behaviors?" The same type of questioning can consolidate and expedite the process of change. Moving from the behaviors to the beliefs one might ask: "Given what you just did, how does that influence your belief that . . . ?" Moving from beliefs to behaviors one might work to crystallize a new, more functional belief about personal adequacy, and ask, "Given your idea that maybe you are not as inadequate as you feel, what might you do to test that out?"

The following example shows how a case formulation that leads to focusing exclusively on behaviors can be mistaken.

Geoffrey, age 23, was a junior member of a sales team. His job involved much travelling, and he had no experience of intimate relationships. He was socially isolated, and an expert worrier, especially about his future and his health. At the time of starting treatment he was also worried about having (a normal degree of) floaters in his left eye. His initial goal was to improve his ability to relate to people. Maintenance cycles were easy to formulate, as they involved readily recognized avoidance and safety behaviors such as refusing invitations, not expressing his feelings or making suggestions, and never talking about himself and his feelings. These safety behaviors served to maintain his social isolation. Geoffrey was highly motivated to change and courageously took many risks involving facing the situations he had feared and avoided, and dropping his safety behaviors. He predicted that others would reject his ideas if he showed more initiative at work, and still attempted to do so. He experimented with being more assertive. All this work was designed specifically to provide opportunities for testing his predictions, and when these proved to be unfounded it was expected that his anxiety would decline. However, despite achieving some of his goals for increased social contact, his anxiety remained as high as ever.

At this stage, his therapist tried to achieve a deeper understanding of his "felt sense" of vulnerability and discovered that reformulating his difficulties in terms of beliefs, instead of in terms of maintenance cycles perpetuated by fear and avoidance, opened up new routes to change. Discussions revealed that Geoffrey held the idiosyncratic belief that the floaters in his eye meant that he had lost his youth. He believed that unless the floaters disappeared his life would be over before it had begun. This understanding led to a shift in the focus of therapy: to thinking about the meaning to Geoffrey of being a young person (his beliefs and assumptions), and about what he wanted to do while he was young; about how he wanted to live his life now so as to be able to expect a different kind of future (his behaviors). This clarified his priorities, and many behavioral changes followed, including seeking a new job that allowed him more free time. The impact on him of the floaters diminished, and he noticed them less. Being clearer about his priorities did not remove his anxiety entirely, but it enabled him to accept and to tolerate the fear better, and to move forward in ways that to him felt significant.

The second example illustrates what may happen if the therapeutic work focuses on beliefs at the expense of behaviors.

Liz was 32, and a single parent with two children. She was fearful of going out to work, but in serious financial need. She had panic attacks at night and a nervous, anxious demeanor. She wanted to talk in treatment about the emotional and practical neglect that she had experienced as a child; about physical abuse at the hands of her former partner, her fear of entering new relationships, and issues concerning mistrust. Her beliefs about herself, about others, and about the world were all highly relevant and easy to talk about. She developed a good relationship with her therapist and started to feel more valued and worthwhile during sessions, a feeling that did not last once she returned home. She made no practical changes at this stage of therapy, and her anxiety remained high—until the behavioral aspects of her difficulties, such as her reluctance to go out on her own, or to seek work, were brought to the fore. As these were linked with her beliefs, for example about the hostility of others and her own inadequacies, she started to explore and to make behavioral changes, and also—slowly but surely—to construct a new and more functional set of beliefs.

It may be worth noting that it can be easy to make this mistake. Liz's belief systems were readily understood, and responses to the distress caused by her experiences of neglect and abuse were readily elicited. At the same time, her reaction to focusing on the behaviors was that it made little difference: just "a drop in the ocean." To her and to her therapist, they seemed at first less important than the underlying beliefs. However, working on beliefs without anchoring the work in behavioral change and experiment may not only be less productive, but also run the risk of losing the way: of getting lost in conceptual hyperspace. In our experience, patients' expectations are often of talking in general about their problems rather than focusing down on details of specific events. Working only at the more abstract level prevents therapists from acquiring the discipline of unpicking and understanding specific mechanisms and sequences that contribute to the persistence of anxiety.

A third example illustrates how some behavioral patterns can produce vicious circles that are especially difficult to break, as if they "get you coming and going." Again it helps to work on the behaviors and on associated underlying beliefs.

Nadim suffered from avoidant personality disorder. He became extremely anxious when interacting with others and went to great lengths to hide what he was really like. He spent hours preparing himself to go out: washing repeatedly, trying on different clothes, combing his hair, and so on. He was unable to answer his door-bell in case people would find him unprepared—and unprotected—and conclude that he was "downright weird." Sometimes he dressed in a sober and conventional way, hoping that would make him acceptable. On other occasions he dressed flam-boyantly, in ways that he thought would be eye-catching and attractive. In either case, the reactions of others to him confirmed his beliefs about being weird and confirmed that he should never be seen "unprepared," without his protective clothing (or mask). A positive response indicated that his disguises worked and should be continued. A negative response suggested that his disguises were not sufficiently successful, so he needed to work harder on them. Nadim described another situation that demonstrated the pervasiveness of such a process. When travelling to therapy Nadim said he had caught the eye of the bus conductor as he paid for his ticket. Because the bus conductor looked at him, Nadim concluded that the bus conductor must think he was weird. Then the bus conductor looked away, and he came to the same conclusion, this time because the bus conductor (apparently) could no longer look at him.

In such cases it is extremely difficult to achieve any lasting change without work-ing on beliefs and behaviors together. The main strategy was to link all types of dressing-up behaviors preparatory to meeting people to his beliefs about himself and to the assumptions that followed from those beliefs. He believed he was weird and made various assumptions about how he should behave to keep his weirdness hidden from others, hence the protective behaviors. The first useful step for Nadim came from working on his beliefs, and throwing doubt on his criteria for acceptability (not being weird) and for judging weirdness. Until this time these had been largely derived from internal events (his feelings about how he came across to others; his conclusions about the significance of looking, or not looking at him). He found abstract discussions about acceptability, weirdness, being different from others and unique, and about being him-self fascinating, and provocative. He began to observe others closely and to take note of the way they responded to each other. He started to doubt his previous beliefs and became curious about trying out ways of "being himself." Behavioral changes followed and provided the data for more objective judgments about what others find acceptable (or not).

So in cases such as these, when comorbidity and complexity make straightforward methods hard to apply, it helps to have both slices of bread in the sandwich, and to make clear links between them. Keeping the specific behaviors and the more general beliefs in mind helps to make the treatment of complex cases into a coherent whole, and in this way it contributes much to the work of case formulation. Theoretically, given the hierarchical way in which cognitions are represented, the sooner beliefs are included in the formulation, the more efficient the work will be. It is even possible that drawing explicit conclusions in terms of beliefs would expedite treatment in more straightforward cases for which conventional methods currently suggest it is sufficient to focus on more proximal maintaining factors. Explicitly identifying beliefs would help to ensure that specific interventions are linked to general sources of difficulty and thus be more likely to lead to generalization.

Using the Case Formulation

A case formulation that fits with theory provides hypotheses about how to change. It suggests which thoughts, assumptions, and beliefs should be worked on, which reactions serve the purpose of protection or safety seeking and prevent adaptive change, which are the facts and which are the hypotheses. It shows where the gaps are and provides ideas about problems that may arise during treatment, and about how the problems fit together, form patterns of relating to others, link up with past experiences, and so on. The case formulation becomes a source of fruitful questions such as "What does this suggest about how to change? What do you want to do differently? What do you predict would happen if . . . ?"

Engaging the Patient in Teamwork

A formulation that belongs only to the therapist is potentially far less useful than one that is worked on together, drawn up collaboratively, and owned by the patient. It is therefore essential that therapists learn how to use the Socratic method and guided discovery to derive their formulations (using questions such as those listed in Figure 3.2). For example, they should learn how to explain their ideas about formulation simply, in ordinary language; practice explaining the ideas behind cognitive therapy to those who know nothing about them; search for and respond to doubts and reservations; and find out how patients already understand their difficulties. The work of formulation is nearly always a matter of *reformulation*, as few people experience persistent problems and difficulties without trying to make sense of them in their own way. So it is important to explore these ideas and to take account of what is right and what is mistaken about them when developing a new version. It is also important to search for a language that has meaning for a patient, possibly using and adapting the terms already used, and listening carefully for signs of cultural and linguistic variation. Metaphors can be extremely helpful, provided that they work for the patient (see also Chapters 2 and 9). For example, one patient described his anxiety as a product of building a rigid building on a fault line and likened treatment to a way of rebuilding the framework for his life with the flexibility needed to withstand an earthquake. Using the language of increasing flexibility helped him to be more creative in his response to difficulties, and also more relaxed in the face of the unknown. Asking about rigidity helped him to understand his symptoms of high anxiety and to respond more flexibly to them.

Checking Out What Has Been Understood

Understanding of abstract ideas, such as those involved in formulation work, may be more apparent than real, especially for concrete thinkers, who may be more confused than helped by using metaphors. Again it is essential to listen carefully to the language used. This is especially useful when facing obstacles to progress despite having a case formulation that seems (to the therapist) to fit. Asking the person to explain how he or she understands the theory of cognitive therapy, and how it fits for him or her often reveals misunderstandings or reservations that could be interfering with progress, and it may also reveal mistakes the therapist has made concerning theories or facts, for instance, about the weight or relevance to be given to a past event (being teased or bullied), or to a particular past experience (fainting in public).

Including Positive and Functional Factors in the Case Formulation

It is important to formulate positive and functional factors at all levels, including beliefs and assumptions. One option is to draw up functional maintenance circles using material from another aspect of the patient's life. Paula, for example (p. 61), put much energy into keeping in touch with her girlfriends by telephone and by e-mail when she found it hard to travel, and their responses gave her a sense of belonging. She was also a tidy and organized person, and on better days at work could achieve a lot in a short time. Creating a more positive context for the discussion in therapy changes the perspective from which problems are seen and may also enable both parties to identify and draw on sources of strength or resilience that they might otherwise have overlooked during the problem-focused interactions that tend to predominate in the therapy room. Such work also carries metamessages about someone's strength or resilience; about that person's ability to be creative, to solve problems, and to change.

Communicating Your Ideas about Formulation Carefully

On the receiving end of a case formulation (especially if provided as a monologue) a person can feel that he or she has been summed up, or judged, or that his or her defenses have been "seen through," or penetrated. Theoretical underpinnings of cognitive therapy suggest that patterns of thinking, feeling, and behaving develop because they served a purpose. They made sense at the time (not trusting anyone, operating in hypervigilant, self-protective mode, for instance) and the pattern became fixed because—to a degree at least—it worked. Again it helps to make the formulation collaboratively with many pauses for reflection and feedback, so that doubts and reservations can be explored. Presenting the ideas Socratically makes the process interactive and stops therapists "talking in paragraphs" (or even in whole chapters). Use the language of "trying to make sense" rather than of "giving a formulation," or telling someone how their experiences fit with a preconceived model. Ask yourself, "Will I be heard?" Ask patients whether there are aspects of their problem or layers of their diffi-

---

1. **Consider the relationship**. Can you collaborate? Do you have sufficient mutual trust? Is the patient able to handle relevant feelings? Can you?

2. **Coping**. What support systems are available? Is this person skilled at keeping himself (and others) safe? Is self-harm or suicidality an issue to consider?

3. **Understanding**. Do you have an idea about what links with what? About how the theories might apply? Is this person able to make links? How does he or she currently understand his or her difficulties? Will this interfere with entertaining a different possibility? Can you see how to search for information that might distinguish different possibilities? (e.g., concerning the genetic, physiological, social, and psychological contributions to the problem?)

4. **Level of metacognitive awareness**. Can this person reflect on his or her experiences (including thoughts, feelings, and behaviors) or is the person caught up in subjectivity, without being able to stand back and think about his or her own experiences (and those of others)? Can the person distinguish thoughts and feelings? Can he or she consider the possibility that there are alternative ways of seeing things—different perspectives? (For more on this, see Chapter 4.)

FIGURE 3.9. The question of readiness.

culty that they have not fully described. Consider whether there are things you should not share, or things that a patient may not be ready for. Obviously this too is a matter for clinical judgment, and some of the parameters to consider are listed in Figure 3.9.

Risks to Watch Out For

Perhaps the main risk is that people may "hear" a case formulation as confirmation of their beliefs, rather than as a way of understanding their origins and their contributions to the maintenance of problems. Sharing a (longitudinal) formulation can be risky for someone with a strong habit of self-blame ("I knew it was all my fault"), and sometimes also for people who habitually blame others and find it hard to accept responsibility ("Everything would be alright if only they would pay attention to what I say . . . love me the way I need . . . apologize as if they meant it"). As Padesky (1993a) pointed out, preconceived ideas may operate like a prejudice: People can hear confirmation of their own ideas even when it was not intended, and they can also ignore, deflect, or distort information that is inconsistent with them (as shown in the Mental Crusher, Figure 3.4). Counterschematic information may be screened out (not attended to); it may not be stored or linked with other related information, and it is difficult to recall, or easy to forget. Repetition may help, and wider psychological principles suggest that the more people work with such information, for example, to identify it, search for it, label it, fit it into current understanding, and make meaningful use of it, for example, as a basis for behavioral experiments, the more likely it is that they will be able to recall it when they need to.

Adapting According to the Stage of Treatment

At first the emphasis is on communicating that it is possible to make sense of the patient's current predicament: on giving information and on seeking a way of understanding problems. This understanding then provides a rationale for the selection of specific interventions. At this stage formulation work can also enhance engagement, collaboration, and motivation and provide a practice ground for giving and getting feedback. It illustrates well the explicit style of cognitive therapy. During the middle phases of treatment the formulation provides a tool to help therapists check and recheck that the work is on track, makes sense, and is likely to assist in reaching the desired ends. The formulation may need fine-tuning or it may need radical change to fit with new findings and observations. It can be used to identify gaps in understanding and to help anticipate and predict difficulties in the therapeutic relationship, process issues, setbacks or future problems, and so on. If the process of change falters or becomes stuck, the formulation can be used as a source of questions to help in the process of troubleshooting. Toward the end of therapy it can serve as a template for making a blueprint, or summary of the ideas learned during treatment (as illustrated in Chapter 10). It can guide future work to be carried on by the patient once therapy has ended and pinpoint future vulnerabilities and ways of dealing with them. It may indicate that some problems have not been solved during therapy and help both parties to consider whether similar methods could potentially help. If so, it is valuable to summarize the cognitive approach parsimoniously, using ordinary language: for example, "First work out how you see things, then search for new perspectives, and test them out in practice." This makes sense of the "unfinished business" in familiar terms and clarifies implications that follow from that.

Drawing metaconclusions is another possibility. For instance, the fact that someone has been able to use cognitive therapy, and has changed her behavior, become more confident, become able to understand things differently, and so on, tells that person something about herself. Work out what implications this has for her and for her future, remembering that the metamessage of formulation work is not that there is a solution to every problem, or that cognitive therapy will resolve all difficulties, but that it is possible and useful to understand what is going on—to make sense of it. Formulation work helped Paula draw the conclusion that "It's not that everything is a problem. There's one problem and that's not being confident." By the end of therapy she knew that that could change, bit by bit. It may be more useful, and consistent with a broad understanding of anxiety problems and the reasons for them, to acknowledge that difficulties, worries, and anxieties will always occur in the future, and that fostering the ability to adapt or roll with the punches may be the best that any of us can expect to do in a world full of uncertainties (see Chapter 9).

CONCLUSION

This chapter has made reference to numerous clinical skills involved in the process of producing clear, theoretically sound, hypothetical, and useful case formulations. In summary, it is argued that these can be held together by using the principle of parsimony to ensure that the formulation is kept as simple as possible, and by paying close attention to each person's "felt sense" of vulnerability, or belief system. A new strategy for therapists, applying the sandwich principle combines use of these principles with a practical, down-to-earth focus on changing specific behaviors. Using their clinical judgment, and the two essential skills of abstraction and selection, therapists can discover how to use the work of formulation to provide much more than a mere template for treatment. Sensitive formulation work helps people to make sense of complex problems, and it also enables patients to recognize and to build on their strengths, to collaborate, give accurate feedback, reflect anew on their experiences, and to make new plans.

These principles and ideas are intended to help therapists in the task of making sense (in theoretical terms) when faced with unusual, atypical, or complex forms of anxiety, and to use their understanding to build their interventions on reasonable foundations. More detailed ideas about specific aspects of treatment are provided in all of the remaining chapters. It is difficult to help people who suffer from complex anxiety disorders, and therefore problems will continue to arise. One of the best sources of solutions comes from the processes of formulation, and of reformulation. All of the work involved, including the implicit or metamessages delivered on the way, may contribute. Retaining a questioning attitude toward a formulation, to the uses made of it, and to the work surrounding it helps to guide a search for solutions. It also serves as a reminder that, when it comes to formulation work, patients as well as therapists have much to contribute. They may even know best.

FOUR

Decentering from Thoughts
Achieving Objectivity

Consider for a moment. If you were 100% convinced that leaving your house meant certain death, how would you react to a therapist who suggested you take a trip to the local supermarket? If you knew for a fact that the pain in your stomach was a sign of cancer, would you be willing to abandon your search for extensive medical tests and embark on psychological treatment? If the idea that your thoughts could kill those dear to you was entirely credible to you, would you be prepared to simply let them come and go? If you fully believed that to experience emotion would leave you forever a weeping heap on the floor, would you risk turning toward painful feelings and memories? If, on the other hand, you were able to accept, difficult as it might be, that your beliefs were ideas you had acquired along the way, learned opinions based on earlier experience, but with no current real-world validity—what then?

Our task as cognitive therapists is to help patients move toward exploring alternative perspectives and actively engaging in the process of change. This is difficult when they fully identify with their own ideas: that is, when they see them as reflections of objective truth, as in the examples outlined above. The absence of metacognitive awareness (the capacity to experience thoughts as thoughts, events in the mind) can make it difficult for patients even to contemplate the possibility of change and indeed can block their willingness to engage in therapy at all. How can you change something that is objectively true, a simple matter of fact?

Working to enhance metacognitive awareness, right from the outset, can encourage engagement even in patients who are at first strongly convinced that what they think is true. It introduces an element of doubt about the validity of old, habitual thoughts, assumptions, and beliefs and potentially illuminates the cognitive mechanisms by which patients unwittingly keep problems going (e.g., screening out information that does not fit the prevailing view). Encouraging patients at least to *entertain* the idea that even powerful, emotionally charged beliefs may be more a matter of opinion than of fact allows them to begin the process of achieving distance from their own thinking. This goes beyond pure case formulation: It involves not only understanding in a general sense how the system works, its elements, and their interconnections, but being able to observe the system in action, moment by moment, from a distance, without getting caught up in the moving machinery. This in turn opens up the possibility of moving toward "So that's what's going on" or "Here I go again," rather than "This is me" or "This is the way it is." We now look in more detail at practical ways of facilitating this process.

THE METACOGNITIVE PERSPECTIVE

In the last 10–15 years, the development of cognitive therapy has been shaped by a growing interest in examining and changing people's relationships to internal experiences, including physical sensations and symptoms (panic, health anxiety, chronic fatigue), emotions (e.g., Leahy, 2002), and cognitive phenomena such as worry, rumination and intrusive thoughts, images, and memories. In each case, the suggestion is that difficulties are maintained by persistent misinterpretations of the significance of internal states and events (in the case of anxiety, "fear of fear"; Rachman & Bichard, 1988), and by the unhelpful behaviors that these engender. These "safety-seeking behaviors" (Salkovskis, 1991) are designed to control problems but in fact paradoxically keep them in place and may indeed exacerbate them. Thus, for example, a person with PTSD might see intrusive memories as a sign of impending loss of control and forcibly suppress them. The person believes that suppression prevents loss of control. In fact, however, suppression ensures that the memories will return with greater frequency and force, whereas the emotional processing necessary for recovery cannot occur (Ehlers & Clark, 2000).

Changing the significance people attach to their own unhelpful ideas (cognitions about cognition, or "metacognition") is central to many contemporary approaches to anxiety disorders. Some use the methods of classical cognitive therapy to question and test metacognitive beliefs, for example, Adrian Wells's metacognitive therapy for GAD (Wells, 1995, 1997, 2000; Wells & Matthews, 1994, 1996), and Paul Salkovskis's approach to OCD (Morrison & Westbrook, 2004; Salkovskis, 1999). Other cognitive approaches have similar objectives in mind but adopt different change methodologies. For example, mindfulness-based cognitive therapy integrates elements of cognitive therapy with intensive practice of mindfulness meditation (Baer, 2003; Ma & Teasdale, 2004; Segal, Williams, & Teasdale, 2002; Teasdale, 2004; Teasdale et al., 2000). Similarly, the capacity to decenter from unhelpful thinking is viewed as foundational in treatments as diverse as dialectical behavior therapy (DBT; Linehan 1993a, 1993b), acceptance and commitment therapy (ACT; Hayes, Strosahl, & Wilson, 1999), and mentalization therapy (Bateman & Fonagy, 2004). These approaches, despite the diversity of their underlying theoretical rationales, share a common goal with cognitive therapy: to teach patients to view their own cognitions as simply mental events and processes, to which they need not attend and on which they need not act.

ASPECTS OF COGNITIVE THERAPY
THAT ENHANCE METACOGNITIVE AWARENESS

Cognitive therapy includes a number of procedures that can be used to promote metacognitive awareness (Moore, 1996). Fennell (2004) suggested that the impact of these might be enhanced if therapists more consciously and systematically used them in such a way as to maximize opportunities for self-observation and self-reflection. This could increase patients' ability to step out of automatic pilot, stand back from their convictions, and view them as learned opinions or ideas, rather than identifying with them and experiencing them as reflections of objective truth. They could then begin to observe the workings of their own minds with interest, curiosity, and compassion rather than with fear, self-judgment and distress ("to get inquisitive about this stuff," as one patient put it). Initially, such a perspective may only be glimpsed momentarily, and with many patients (especially with those whose difficulties are long-standing and entrenched) achieving it can be a slow process to which sessions return again and again.

The Therapeutic Relationship

When anxious, patients believe that the dangers they confront are real and potentially damaging. As a result, they approach situations that to an outsider would appear trivial with genuine terror. A relatively calm, unshockable, compassionate guide helps to create the confidence that things may not be quite as they appear, and that change is possible. Ideally, the cognitive therapist embodies the spirit of collaborative empiricism, and in so doing fosters a similar approach on the part of the patient—tuned to approach rather than to avoidance, inquiring, adaptable, and kind. We acknowledge that, in practice, attaining this ideal can be hard. Like us, readers will no doubt from time to time have lost their way, told rather than asked, backed off from necessary experiments, felt like the blind leading the blind, become exasperated or hopeless, wondered if what they are doing was remotely helpful, and encountered many other doubts and stumbling blocks. Nonetheless, as we have emphasized elsewhere, the clinical literature on cognitive therapy provides us with a template toward which we can helpfully aspire. It places technical cognitive therapy interventions firmly in the context of a warm, empathic, collaborative therapeutic relationship, which facilitates learning and creates a safe space within which patients can explore fresh perspectives and experiment with new ways of thinking and acting. The therapist's confidence that there may be other ways of looking at things, that progress can be made, that difficulties and setbacks can be part of the learning process if approached with an investigative mind, and with flexibility and creative problem solving, help to foster similar confidence in the patient.

More specifically, therapists can model the decentered perspective that they would like patients to adopt. They can, for example, explicitly describe and name unhelpful cognitive processes they observe in patients and map their impact (e.g., "That sounds like worry. Could that be your old 'better safe than sorry' assumption coming on line? How does that feel? What does it incline you to do?"). They would also do well to reflect on their own responses, fine-tuning awareness of assumptions and beliefs activated in therapy and the thoughts, emotions, and behavior that follow from them (Bennett-Levy, 2006; Schön, 1983, 1987). This is particularly important with complex cases (especially perhaps when anxiety is comorbid with personality disorder) where process issues are more likely to come to the fore (Beck, Freeman, Davis, & Associates, 2004, Chapter 5).

Assessment Instruments

Standard questionnaires (e.g., measuring key cognitions or safety-seeking behaviors) can prompt recognition of aspects of experience that contribute to the problem, but of which patients lost in anxiety may have been barely aware. One patient, for example, was unaware how much effort she put into disguising her true thoughts and feelings for fear of rejection until she completed a questionnaire assessing social safety-seeking behaviors (Wells, 1997). Items on the questionnaire highlighted what pains she took to avoid eye contact with people who looked concerned or sympathetic, monitored her tone of voice, and tried to "look normal," that is, untroubled, cheerful, vivacious.

Formulation

As we discussed in Chapter 3, cognitive-behavioral case formulations delineate the historical processes through which problems develop and the recurrent sequences of thoughts, emotions, body states, and behaviors that maintain them. Sharing the formulation, provided it is sensitively handled, provides an opportunity for the patient to move toward "This is what I have learned" and "This makes sense, given my experiences," rather than "This is how things really are."

Treatment Rationale

The cognitive therapy rationale implies that change is possible, and that there are effective ways of bringing it about. This broad message is an important part of awakening hope in patients whose problems may seem confusing and entrenched. It is not necessary for them to be immediately convinced that all will be well. Rather, the key thing is to encourage a willingness to be open minded and to experiment.

Written Materials

Written materials such as copies of formulation flowcharts, session summaries, handouts, and the like offer opportunities to reflect on and consolidate work done in session. Printed handouts and self-help texts also communicate an important message: "I'm not alone" and "It's not just me."

"Signposting" and Decentering Questions

Therapists can use guided discovery to foster metacognitive awareness by "signposting" key cognitions and highlighting their connections to problem development and persistence. Exploratory and synthesizing questions (Padesky, 1993b) can be used as prompts to help patients to relate current work to the broader formulation (e.g., "How does this relate to the ideas we identified earlier about your responsibility for others?"; "How might what we are working on today connect up with that sense of impending doom you talked about when we first met?"; "Where would this fit in our formulation flowchart?"; "What's this an example of?"; "Whose voice was that speaking?"). Similar questions ensure that work on specific instances is related back to more general beliefs and assumptions (e.g., "What are the implications of this experiment for your idea that physical symptoms always have a sinister explanation?"), and conversely that work on broader issues is firmly grounded in day-to-day experiences (e.g., "What could you do this week to test out your new rule about balancing pleasing others against your own needs?"). This is the sandwich principle we developed in Chapter 3 (p. 64), through which the specific can be repeatedly related to the general, and vice versa. Finally, therapists' sensitivity to the operation of old patterns can help patients to become aware of these as they occur (e.g., "What happened just then? Did you notice what immediately came to mind when we began to talk about venturing out of your comfort zone?" and "I noticed that when I said that, you looked away. What was going on there?").

Developing Day-to-Day Awareness of Recurrent Cognitive Patterns

Record sheets such as the Dysfunctional Thoughts Record (DTR; Beck et al., 1979), the record of behavioral experiments (see Chapter 6), and schema worksheets tune in patients to noticing unhelpful thinking as it occurs in everyday life. They help people to recognize situations in which their personal vulnerabilities are triggered, and to identify emotional and physical reactions associated with different cognitions, and behavioral responses that contribute to problem maintenance or promote change. Patients sometimes remark that self-monitoring with the help of such structured record sheets reduces their sense of distress and confusion, in that it takes the problem "out of their heads" onto the page, where they can take a step back and begin the process of disengagement ("Oh, look, there it is again"). Later in therapy, this in itself can be enough to nip in the bud a distressing train of thought.

Relapse Prevention

It is possible that old systems are never, so to speak, "deleted from the hard disk," but rather that treatment provides people with an elaborated repertoire of alternative responses that, with repeated practice, become prepotent. With anxiety, as with depression, the possibility that old patterns of cognition will recur, given the right circumstances, needs to be taken into account. The therapy "blueprint" or learning summary and action plan (see Chapter 10) encourages patients to reflect on how their problems developed, what kept them going, what they have learned in therapy, what might lead to a setback for them, and how they would deal with any setback that did occur.

SPECIFIC METHODS FOR ENHANCING METACOGNITIVE AWARENESS

In addition to using the therapeutic relationship and working systematically to enhance the impact of familiar elements of classical cognitive therapy, a number of specific interventions can be employed that directly facilitate metacognitive awareness. Readers will recognize that some of these have already been introduced in Chapter 3, where we emphasized their role in formulation. Here, however, the emphasis is rather on how to use them to encourage detached awareness of and distance from problematic cognitive and behavioral patterns.

The "Prejudice Model"

Padesky's (1993a) prejudice model, originally designed as a framework for recognizing cognitive and behavioral processes that contribute to low self-esteem (effectively, a prejudice against the self), provides a helpful template for investigating information-processing biases in a much broader range of problem areas including the beliefs that fuel anxiety (e.g., "Stress is dangerous," "People are hostile," "I can't cope"). Padesky suggested asking patients to call to mind a person they know (either personally or through history or the media) who has a prejudice with which they do not agree. Identifying another person's prejudice (rather than working on one of their own) contributes to distancing; it is generally much easier to notice the flaws in another person's argument and their unhelpful little ways than it is to be aware of the same difficulties in oneself. Patients can then be asked to describe:

- How the person they have selected reacts when they meet someone who fits the prejudice (e.g., saying "I told you so" and feeling smug).
- How they react when they meet someone who does *not* fit the prejudice (i.e., by what means they keep the prejudice intact—for example, failing to notice, saying that this is the exception that proves the rule, avoiding).
- What the person would need to do to change (e.g., recognizing the prejudice as a prejudice, deliberately seeking out examples that contradict it).
- What would make change difficult (including not only cognitive biases and behavioral precautions, but also environmental and interpersonal pressures and the force of early learning).

This exploratory procedure is then linked back to therapy ("Why are we discussing this?" and "What's the connection between this and the issues you and I have been working on?"). Thus a process of guided discovery helps patients to become more aware of how perception, interpretation, and memory can all be skewed by preexisting, ingrained ideas (believed to reflect objective fact), and to see how developing a more balanced point of view might be possible, while appreciating that it may not be easy to achieve.

Theory 1, Theory 2

Paul Salkovskis (1996) stated: "The most effective way of changing a misinterpretation . . . is to help the person come up with an alternative, less threatening interpretation of his or her experience" (p. 58). This is exactly the purpose of "Theory 1, Theory 2." This intervention has been helpfully elaborated in relation to health anxiety (e.g., Warwick & Salkovskis, 2001). It can be readily applied to other anxiety disorders, and indeed to a wider range of problematic beliefs including transdiagnostic issues such as low self-esteem (see Chapter 8). Patients with health anxiety often enter psychological treatment with serious doubts about its relevance to their needs. Indeed, they may firmly believe that it has nothing to offer, given their conviction that they are (or will be) physically ill (Theory 1). It follows that the problem is their state of health, not their psychology, and consequently what they need is medical attention. When treatment begins, Theory 1 is likely to be strongly held by the patient, but the therapist (provided proper medical checks have been carried out) will probably be more skeptical about its validity. Theory 2 in health anxiety is the alternative idea that the patient is in fact perfectly well, or at least no less healthy than anyone else, but that she or he *believes* that she or he is ill; that is, the problem is not physical ill health, but the patient's thinking. The patient does not need to accept this idea at all to begin with, and indeed is likely to be quite skeptical about it, or anxious about abandoning Theory 1 in case it proves to be true. What is necessary is the willingness to temporarily suspend judgment and to engage in an extended experiment with psychological treatment to discover which of the two theories better fits careful observation of day-to-day experience. If at the end of (say) 3 months the patient remains convinced that the real problem is illness, then she or he can always return to further medical consultations. (A range of possible Theories 1 and 2, relevant to different anxiety disorders, can be found in Table 4.1.)

Early in treatment, it may be difficult or impossible for a patient to articulate Theory 2 herself, though sometimes she can begin to identify an alternative to an old belief in response to questions such as, "If this were not so, how would you like it to be?" The ideal is for the patient to discover a possible Theory 2 through guided discovery, but it may be necessary initially for the therapist to make direct suggestions. These should be tentative and respectful of the patient's right to see things differently. For example, in the case of a patient with emotional avoidance (see Chapter 7), the therapist might proceed somewhat as follows—though interspersing plentiful opportunities for the patient to question, comment and disagree (perhaps as indicated below), not as a lecture:

TABLE 4.1. Examples of Theory 1 and Theory 2 in Different Problem Areas

Problem area	Example of Theory 1	Possible Theory 2
Panic disorder	"I am about to die/go mad/lose control, etc."	"These sensations are quite normal, but *I believe* that I am about to die, etc."
Health anxiety	"I am ill."	"I am as fit as anyone else, but *I believe* I am ill."
Social anxiety	"I must meet high standards as a social being in order to be acceptable to others."	"In fact, most people will accept me for what I am, but *I believe* I have to put on a show."
Specific phobia	"This thing is dangerous."	"This thing is harmless—I have just learned to see it as dangerous."
OCD	"I am a danger to others."	"I am a harmless, and indeed careful and kindly person, but *I believe* that I am a danger to others."
GAD	"My life is full of things that might go wrong and, if they do, I might not be able to cope."	"I am a person who worries a lot and finds it difficult to be comfortable with uncertainty."
PTSD	"I am in danger."	"The trauma, and my failure to process it properly, has made me feel as if I am in danger."

"OK, so your conviction at the moment is that emotions are dangerous, and indeed that if you were to allow yourself fully to experience what you feel, you would simply collapse. Is that right? [*Feedback*] OK, let's call that Theory 1. Now, just for a moment, let's suppose that there might be another way of looking at this. Supposing, just for the sake of argument, emotions were in fact a normal part of being human, but that you had learned along the way to *believe* that they were dangerous and have to be suppressed. [*Feedback*] Let's call that idea Theory 2. Now, if Theory 1 is true, then the real problem is your dangerous emotions—what you need to do here is to learn to keep them firmly under control, even when the going gets rough, as it has recently. [*Feedback*] But if Theory 2 is true (which I can see you feel pretty doubtful about [*Feedback*], then the problem is not your emotions, but your *beliefs* about them. [*Feedback*] If so, then what you need to do is to check out whether these beliefs are actually realistic and helpful, and perhaps to learn to explore and become comfortable with your emotions instead of trying to shove them aside and squash them. [*Feedback*] Our sessions present an opportunity to investigate these two theories, and see which one works best for you. What's your reaction to that idea? [*Feedback*]

The therapist is not attempting to convert the patient to the new perspective (Theory 2) but rather to suggest that there may be more than one way to understand what is going on, and to foster curiosity and flexibility in the patient's mind. The aim is to open the door to situations that offer patients a chance to test out old and new perspectives through direct personal experience (investigative dialogue and behavioral experiments). The specific models and treatment protocols outlined in Chapter 1 provide a wide range of creative interventions designed to investigate and test the ideas specific to different anxiety disorders (see also Chapter 6 in this volume, and Bennett-Levy, Butler, et al., 2004).

Readers can see from Table 4.1 that the content of Theory 1 is largely specific to the problem area under consideration, whereas the content of Theory 2 reflects a strong underlying, transdiagnostic theme: "Experience has taught me to see things in a certain way, and *that* is the real problem." Equally, a common implication follows from Theory 2: "My thoughts, assumptions, and beliefs may be learned opinions rather than reflections of objective reality." This is the essence of metacognitive awareness.

It is worth laying out a patient's Theory 1 and Theory 2 visually, for example, in the two columns shown in the example in Figure 4.1), so that therapist and patient can stand back and look at the different possibilities side by side. This can be done on paper, or on a whiteboard or flipchart. If a whiteboard or flipchart is used, summarizing the discussion on paper allows therapist and patient to keep copies to reflect on and develop further if they wish to do so.

"Vicious Flowers"

The "vicious flower" captures in visual form the way that a central concern or preoccupation can prompt unhelpful cognitions and behaviors, which in turn feed back into and strengthen it (see Chapter 2, Figure 2.1, and Chapter 8, Figure 8.1, for more examples). In particular, it shows clearly how strategies intended to solve the problem (e.g., safety-seeking behaviors) may in fact inadvertently keep it going. The "vicious flower"

Theory 1	Theory 2
Emotions are dangerous and must be controlled at all costs.	Emotions are a normal part of being human, but
That is:	I have learned to see them as dangerous.
The problem is my emotions, and the fact that they might get out of hand. If this happened, no one would want to know me.	*That is:*
What I need to do is:	The problem is my ideas about emotion, not my emotions in themselves.
Learn to control them better, even under difficult circumstances.	*What I need to do is:*
	Allow myself to be human and have the same emotions everyone else does.

FIGURE 4.1. Theory 1 and Theory 2: An example.

is so called because the arrows representing maintenance factors look like the petals of a flower, whose center is the concern under consideration (see Figures 4.2 and 4.3a for examples). The centrifugal arrows show how the central concern leads to a range of cognitive and behavioral responses, including specific interpretations (negative automatic thoughts), cognitive processes (e.g., catastrophizing, worry, rumination, hypervigilance), and behaviors such as avoidance, safety-seeking behaviors, and behaviors that have an adverse impact on the patient's environment (especially the interpersonal environment) such as aggression, substance misuse, or withdrawal. The centripetal arrows show how, paradoxically, these in fact maintain and reinforce the central concern. In therapy, the task is then to use cognitive and behavioral methods to dismantle the petals so that the central issue no longer receives sustenance and may indeed be fatally weakened. The beauty of the "flower" format is that it provides a memorable shorthand for what may be quite complex processes and is thus highly portable and easy to call to mind even under stress. It can also be put into its developmental context by adding a stem and a root (see Chapter 2, Figure 2.1, for a generic example).

Figure 4.2 shows the case of Charlie, who came for help with obsessional ruminations, compounded by social evaluative concerns, occasional panic attacks, and recurrent depression (sometimes profound enough for him to contemplate suicide). He did well with cognitive therapy, in particular realizing that he could safely afford to let obsessional thoughts come and go because they had no real significance and there was no need to act on them. However, he asked for further help about 18 months later because, after a period of feeling happy and confident, he had begun to experience low mood and physical symptoms of anxiety for which he felt there was no real reason, and had begun to worry that the whole cycle was starting up again. Charlie and his therapist spent a session carefully exploring his reactions to signs of physiological arousal and low mood and examined the impact of these on his sense that inexplicable anxiety and low mood were dangerous. It emerged that, as soon as he noticed a shift in his emotional state for which he could not easily account, a number of reactions fed his mounting distress. Encapsulating these in a "vicious flower" (Charlie liked the absurdity of the term) helped him to see how initial discomfort spiraled into something more severe and put him in a better position to observe this in action, to "press the pause button," and to respond to normal day-to-day fluctuations in mood without overreacting.

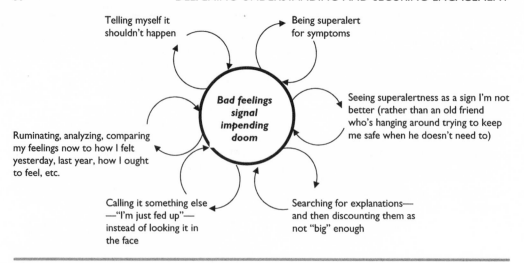

FIGURE 4.2. Charlie's "vicious flower."

"Virtuous Flowers"

A similar format can be used to map out alternatives to old, unhelpful patterns and carries the same benefits (individually tailored, simple, portable, memorable). Figure 4.3a shows the "vicious flower" of Vera, who came for help with what appeared to be a fairly straightforward specific phobia. It soon became clear in therapy that this was in fact only one element in a more complex picture, maintained by a central sense of being bad, pathetic, and responsible when things went wrong. This derived from a complete lack of sympathy in her family—indeed they still would not take her phobia seriously or even acknowledge its reality and the impact it had on her life. As a consequence she felt embarrassing, stupid, and uncared for. The "vicious flower" vividly captured her current sense of entrapment.

She and her therapist then together developed a "virtuous flower" (Figure 4.3b), with possible alternatives to her central beliefs at the center, and ideas for how she might experiment with operating differently in the petals. The patient loved the "virtuous flower"—which she called her "compassionate flower"—as it encouraged a "warm glow" of hope. At follow-up, she commented on its value as a framework for the continuing challenge of changing long-held beliefs: "Has remained a useful reference point to be added to and used regularly to reinforce the compassionate and positive feelings about my behaviors. However when mood is low I don't believe the compassionate flower to be true and struggle to relate it to myself. However, I think it is a great tool which is a brilliant visual aid and a good concept to keep practicing with when I am low, as it's not complicated. I still love it!"

The Cognitive Maintaining Cycle

Fennell (1999, 2006) described a self-maintaining cycle of cognitive processes in diagrammatic form, which she suggested contributes to the persistence of negative beliefs about the self, and which could equally be applied to the continuance of other unhelp-

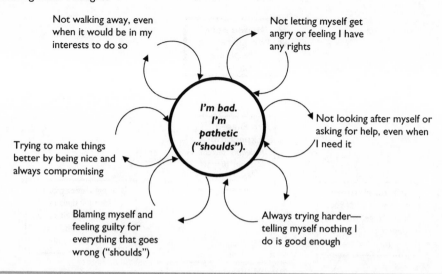

FIGURE 4.3a. Vera's "vicious flower."

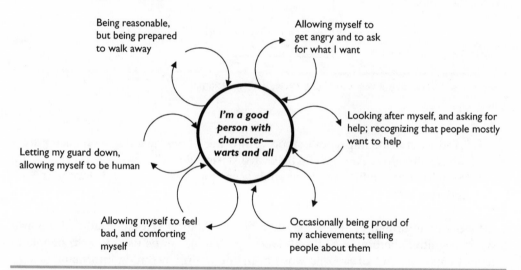

FIGURE 4.3b. Vera's "compassionate flower."

ful ideas (see Figure 4.4). Once a problematic belief has been identified, the cycle can be drawn up with patients through a sequence of exploratory questions:

- "So when you enter a situation relevant to this belief, what do you anticipate?"
- "And once in the situation, what jumps out at you? What do you tend to focus on most?"
- "And what do you make of what you see? What do you take it to mean about you/others/the world/the future?"
- "And afterwards, what do you tend to remember most clearly about the situation? And what tends to be forgotten?"

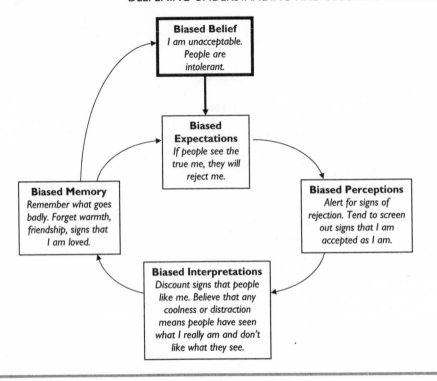

FIGURE 4.4. The cognitive maintaining cycle, with an example.

- "And what is the impact of that on your expectations next time you encounter a similar situation? And on the belief we started with?"
- "So what is this telling us about what keeps the belief going and stops you from updating it?"

Similarly, information about cognitive biases ("logical errors"), outlined in early texts on cognitive therapy (e.g., Burns 1980, pp. 32–43), can be used to help people to tune in to and step out of favorite ways of manipulating incoming information.

Experiments

Small in-session experiments can provide direct experiential evidence of cognitive mechanisms involved in maintaining the status quo. For example, comparing the impact of 2–3 minutes focusing on characteristic worries and concerns with that of 2–3 minutes of externally focused attention ("distraction") can economically demonstrate the link between cognition and emotion. Similarly, the "white bears" experiment (Wegner, Schneider, Carter, & White, 1987) shows how attempting to suppress thoughts actually has the reverse effect. Patients are asked NOT to think about a white bear. If you try this for yourself, you will discover what instantly becomes clear to most patients; paradoxically, the more you try not to think about something, the more it comes to mind. (If you prefer not to think about a green rabbit, consult Rouf et al., 2004, Chapter 2, pp. 31–32.) This is a salutary lesson for patients who have been attempting to control their anxiety by suppressing anxious thoughts (or images or memories) and can helpfully be followed by a homework assignment to be carried out before the next session, and consisting of just allowing thoughts to come and go and observing the impact of doing so (usually, contrary to expectation, their frequency drops).

Metaphors, Analogies, and Images

An apt metaphor or analogy, or an image that captures the essence of a difficulty can at once help a person vividly to clarify the feel of a problem and to see it from a different angle (see also Chapters 2 and 5). Charlie, for example, had difficulty accepting the idea that fluctuations in emotional state might result from an accumulation of small stressors rather than necessarily from some major event. This contributed to his concern about relapse because emotional responses to everyday events seemed inexplicable to him. He found a metaphor useful in grasping the idea that small, even apparently trivial, things can have an impact over time: A pile of pebbles, if it is big enough, weighs as much as a boulder. A computer-literate patient described her sense of stress, pressure, and constant worry as being like a computer with so many "windows" open that the machine stops working efficiently, slows down, and eventually freezes. Holding this image in her mind helped her to become aware of when things were building up, and to step out of the system, close some windows, and give herself space to reflect on what was really troubling her. That made it easier for her to tackle it.

Another patient was terrified of losing control and kept everything in her life under as tight a rein as she could manage. This was a huge effort. She found a metaphor and sensory image for an alternative when her young son wanted to go down a water slide at a local amusement park. He was too young to go alone, and there was no one else to take him, so she gave way to his pleading and agreed to keep him company. The first time, she was tightly braced and very uncomfortable, swinging wildly from side to side and convinced that her last hour had come. She was shaking by the time she landed awkwardly in the pool at the bottom of the slide. Needless to say, one go was not enough for her son so, gritting her teeth, she made her way to the top again. This time, for no reason she could identify, she suddenly got the hang of letting go and allowing the water and the design of the slide to carry her to a safe landing. She was astonished to discover a sense of exhilarated liberation. This experience became her template for responding to things being out of her control: "Wheeee!"

Stories

Stories too can be used to illustrate aspects of the cognitive model and to illuminate how problems develop and are maintained. For example, the "dog mess" story (Salkovskis, 1996, p. 48) illustrates with grace and humor how the same event can be interpreted in many different ways, with varying emotional and behavioral consequences. The story describes the reactions of four different people to stepping in dog mess on the way to work. The first tells himself that he is a failure and assumes that his day is ruined. Understandably, he becomes depressed and goes home to bed. The second (prone to anxiety) begins to fret about what he should do—all the options seem to him fraught with potential catastrophe, and he cannot make up his mind. The third instantly blames his neighbors, becomes enraged, and vows revenge. The fourth is a cognitive therapist, who reacts quite differently. The story concludes: "Looking down at his shoes, he smiled broadly, mopped his forehead, and said to himself, 'Well, isn't it good that I remembered to put my shoes on this morning.' "

CONCLUSION

Powerfully convincing negative beliefs, assumptions, and thoughts can block engagement in therapy for patients who are anxious and help to keep them stuck in old fears. In contrast, decentering from habitual cognitive patterns can overcome this disabling obstacle to progress and open the door to the possibility of change. Metacognitive awareness allows painful issues to be placed on the workbench of the mind, opens out a space for observation and reflection, and creates a framework within which specific cognitive-behavioral interventions can be more effectively carried out.

The aim of the various methods described above goes beyond pure mapping of the territory (case formulation). Not only do they imply making sense of experience, but in addition observing as it occurs the operation of beliefs, assumptions, and thoughts from a detached perspective. When this is done, over time, they lose their capacity to compel.

The essence of metacognitive awareness is encapsulated in the following statement made by George W. Bush in 2002 and reported in the United Kingdom's *Guardian* newspaper: "I have opinions of my own, strong opinions. But I don't always agree with them." That is, enhancing metacognitive awareness may not in itself fundamentally alter the *content* of unhelpful patterns of thinking, but it alters the patient's *relationship* to them in such a way that changes in content, and the articulation and testing of fresh perspectives, become possible. That is, it introduces an element of distance or dis-identification that allows patients to recognize old patterns, and to begin the change process by intentionally standing back from them rather than getting drawn in by their pull (i.e., to disagree with them). People can start to say to themselves, "This is an idea that I have," or "There's that old war wound of mine playing up," as opposed to "This is me" or "This is the truth." Rather than viewing themselves and their worlds through the prism of old beliefs, they can view the beliefs themselves through the clear lens of metacognitive awareness.

PART III

FACILITATING EMOTIONAL PROCESSING

"I can see there's no need to worry, but I can't help doing it."
"I know rationally that there's no real danger but I still don't really feel safe."

The clinical dilemmas explored in this part of the book arise during the middle and later phases of treatment. At this stage the combined processes of assessment, formulation, engagement, and decentering have, at least in theory, enabled the patient to start using the methods of cognitive-behavioral therapy to search for new ways of seeing things. However, it can still be hard to achieve profound and lasting change. As the quotations above illustrate, tentative changes in thinking (knowing with the head) may not be reflected in comparable changes in emotion (knowing with the heart). Or the changes that patients make may be transitory, and their hold on them fragile.

In this part of the book we explore in detail two of the most effective methods of achieving "whole person," lasting change, and suggest how clinicians can work more productively to ensure that gains made by their patients are stable. In Chapter 5, "Bringing About Lasting Change at the Deepest Level," common processes underlying different cognitive techniques are considered, in the context of theoretical models of emotional processing. We address more extensively meanings that are encapsulated in memories, or in symbolic representations such as images, metaphors, and dreams and argue that improving skills for working with more emotive material can greatly extend clinicians' therapeutic range. Chapter 6, "Behavioral Experiments and Experiential Learning," addresses the same problem from a different angle, focusing on effective use of enactive methods to build strong links between the cognitive, physiological, affective, and behavioral aspects of anxiety. It highlights the crucial role of learning through direct, personal experience in resolving many clinical difficulties.

As in the other parts of the book, we illustrate solutions to common dilemmas with real clinical examples and clarify the principles on which solutions are based so as to make the ideas readily usable in a wide range of situations.

FIVE

Bringing About Lasting Change at the Deepest Level

Once key "hot" cognitions have been identified (Chapter 2), a formulation has been developed (Chapter 3), and it is clear that the patient is able to recognize that "thoughts are not facts" (Chapter 4), then the cognitive therapist attempts to work with the cognitions, using a variety of techniques, so that they no longer disrupt functioning in everyday life. Some of the problems we encounter at this stage include changing how people think, but not how they feel; achieving a temporary shift but finding that it does not last; and not being able to produce much in the way of change because we have overlooked some of the relevant appraisals, including perhaps those encapsulated in images or memories, as discussed in Chapter 2.

In this chapter we look at the mechanisms thought to underpin emotional processing and consider a range of common and less familiar techniques within this framework. This is with the aim of understanding the common principles involved in bringing about profound and lasting cognitive, emotional, and behavioral change. We provide more detail on methods of working with more emotive, symbolic material, in the form of images, memories, dreams, and metaphors. This is partly to accommodate to situations in which meanings are initially hard to identify, or to put into words. It is also an area where clinicians may feel they would like to extend their range of strategies, without losing sight of the underlying principles of emotional processing and cognitive therapy.

EMOTIONAL PROCESSING

In a seminal article Rachman (1980) addressed the concept of emotional processing. With reference to Freud's description of Anna O. he describes the symptoms of incomplete emotional processing as including intrusive thoughts, images, memories, and nightmares that are "out of proportion, out of context, or simply out of time." Successful emotional processing is defined as "a process whereby emotional disturbances . . .

decline to the extent that other experiences and behaviour can proceed without disruption" (pp. 51–60). In a later paper Rachman (2001) suggested that this process should be relabeled "cognitive-emotional processing," to take account of advances from the cognitive revolution.

Teasdale has also written about emotional processing. Following a review of the literature he suggested the core process involves three components: the old material is activated, and then held in awareness while a wider array of information is accumulated, preferably in a mindful state of awareness, rather than one of mindless emoting (Teasdale, 1999a).

Theories of emotional processing including those described above, together with those arising from models of autobiographical memory, outlined in Chapter 2, point to underlying common components thought to be important for cognitive-emotional processing. These can be summarized as follows:

- Hot material is activated.
- It is explored in detail (see Chapter 2).
- It is held in awareness while new material is activated.
- This is best done in a state of mindful awareness (see Chapter 4).
- A variety of techniques can be employed to secure the new information.
- The effect of successful emotional processing is to bring things into proportion, update old information, and provide a wider context for understanding events.

These same principles are extended to work with nightmares and to other more metaphorical images. We turn next to procedures that make use of the above principles.

SPONTANEOUS COGNITIVE CHANGE AS A RESULT OF SIMPLY EVOKING HOT MATERIAL

In the assessment of anxiety disorders in cognitive therapy we deliberately evoke hot material, and unpack meanings, as described in Chapter 2. This in itself may be therapeutic. Deliberately evoking emotive material is also an important component of many types of behavioral and cognitive treatment interventions.

Examples of therapeutic procedures in which emotive imagery and thoughts are evoked include reliving traumatic memories in PTSD (Foa & Rothbaum, 1998), imaginal desensitization (Wolpe, 1958), imaginal flooding (Stampfl & Levis, 1967), and eye movement desensitization and reprocessing (EMDR; Shapiro, 2001). Negative automatic thoughts, intrusive imagery, and affect can also be evoked by exposure to an actual feared situation. Situational or imaginal exposure may be brief or prolonged, repeated or a single intervention, stable in content or with varying characteristics. The usual effect of exposure to hot material is a decrease in affect and subsequent intrusions, well documented in the behavior therapy literature.

At this point it may be useful to question the common assumption that the effective element of situational or imaginal exposure is habituation. Foa consistently offered a more complex account of the processes necessary for fear reduction and emotional processing (e.g., Foa & Kozak, 1986). She suggested that the "fear structure" must be activated, and information incompatible with pathological elements must be provided: features later echoed in Teasdale's (1999a, 1999b) account.

One of the procedures classically used by Foa's group in the treatment of PTSD involves reliving a traumatic memory, describing it in detail in the first person, present tense, often with the eyes closed to enhance the strength of the experience. Usually significant affect is evoked, which diminishes over time. Writing about this procedure Jaycox (1998) discussed various mechanisms possibly responsible for improvement with imaginal exposure, in addition to habituation. She suggested that these may include introduction of a sense of safety from the therapy environment, opportunities for discrimination between the trauma and other nontraumatic events, the discovery that facing memories does not lead to losing control, and an opportunity to focus on elements of the trauma that have driven negative evaluations, and modify these. Finally, with repetition, a less fragmented, more coherent narrative starts to emerge (Foa, Molnar, & Cashman, 1995). These aspects of "emotional processing" may also be observed on exposure to situational cues, accompanied by spontaneous cognitive change, even without any deliberate "cognitive" interventions.

Our own clinical practice of cognitive therapy has provided many examples demonstrating that when hot material is evoked spontaneous cognitive change can sometimes be observed. Here are some examples:

During therapy for spider phobia the patient suddenly remarked, "I imagined the spider would rush forward, run up my arm, and bite me—but it hasn't moved much at all." Here an image was spontaneously compared with reality.

A patient with a dog phobia had intrusive images that she did her best to suppress. She was asked to let the image come to mind, and describe it fully. She described a horrible image of several dogs attacking her, biting her, and tearing her dress. This image turned out to be a memory of a childhood nightmare. She described how she appeared in the nightmare and then said with palpable relief, "It's not me now! It's when I was seven years old—it's not now." Thus the image (a fragment of memory) acquired its time code and imparted less of a sense of current threat.

Similarly, a patient with PTSD was taken to the hospital where his daughter had died in traumatic circumstances some years before. He was really scared to visit the ward where she died, exclaiming that he was sure she would still be there in the hospital bed. Finally he was persuaded to enter the ward, and soon reappeared, saying, "It is not about now—of course she is not still there!"

After reliving a terrible car crash for the second time a patient remarked that somehow the memory seemed further away. He was aware while recounting the experience that he was safe now, in the therapist's room, and the upsetting scene he was imagining was only a memory.

Allowing a metaphorical image about a difficult situation to arise can help a person appreciate that they have got things out of proportion. A patient was looking after her frail, elderly father and found it an exhausting experience. Her metaphorical image of this was that he was like a powerful eagle and could carry her off to his lonely nest, and even dismember her. Describing this made her laugh, as she appreciated the fact that in fact he had no real power over her any more, and she could find other people to help her look after him, so that she could get on with her own life while maintaining a caring relationship with him.

Spontaneous cognitive change (during or after exposure to hot material) has been observed in many types of treatment. For example, during desensitization one of Wolpe's students observed that upsetting images did not simply fade or become less distressing: Other images and associations might occur, and the original image could undergo changes (Weitzman, 1967). Desensitization may sometimes have provided opportunities for elaboration and contextualization of fragments of upsetting memories, giving them a time code, and a place in autobiographical memory, so that they were no longer evoked by situational cues. However, Rachman (personal communication, September 2005) notes that this is not a commonly reported experience.

Similarly Levis (1980) reported that recovered memories of traumatic experiences sometimes emerge during imaginal flooding. In this treatment (Stampfl & Levis, 1967) the therapist and patient construct imaginary scenarios representing feared stimuli and worst possible outcomes, which the patient then describes as if they were occurring in the present. This occasionally activates memories that may underlie the fearful images. It is possible that if the patient understands the origins of the fear the patient may be helped to make finer discriminations between the past and the present.

Finally, in EMDR the patient is encouraged to hold in mind an image representing the worst aspect of a situation, having first considered how he would like to feel about it. During this process a string of images and memories arise, sometimes moving in a more positive direction. If this does not occur spontaneously further change may be brought about by incorporating more verbal discussion in a process called the "cognitive interweave."

Thus there is some evidence that spontaneous cognitive change can occur if hot material is held in mind during a therapy session. In cognitive therapy this material can be accessed by discussing a recent specific episode, evoking an image, reliving an upsetting memory, or exposing the patient to situational cues and then unpacking the "felt sense" (as described in Chapter 2). Holding hot material in awareness can help the person to see that it is only an image, a memory, or a thought; it may have its roots in the past; and it may not really be indicative of current threat (i.e., there is a metacognitive shift). Inspection of the hot cognition can enable the person to see that it has the wrong time code, is something taken out of context, and is out of proportion when compared with reality. This may also be one of the processes that account for observations made during the practice of mindfulness meditation when some people notice that if they do not struggle with painful thoughts and feelings, but simply turn toward them and allow them to be there while they reflect on their content, they start to fade or change. This is also described as an aspect of the Buddhist practice of insight meditation (Goldstein & Kornfield, 2001).

USING TRADITIONAL COGNITIVE THERAPY TECHNIQUES TO PROMPT FOR CHANGE, BY HOLDING OLD MATERIAL IN MIND WHILE ACCUMULATING MORE INFORMATION

If sufficient cognitive change does not occur spontaneously there are various ways of prompting for it in cognitive therapy. For example, if a person notices that her images, thoughts, and feelings are out of proportion for the current situation she may be asked to reflect on any previous time in her life when she experienced something in a similar way. Making an *emotional bridge* like this (see Chapter 2) may lead back to a particular event in the past, which appears to be coloring the present. Making a link may in itself be therapeutic, in that the person may be struck that her appraisals owe more to past than to present reality, and may subsequently be more motivated to do *behavioral experiments* to discriminate between the two. A small but significant drop in symptom ratings was noted in a study in which links between images and memories were simply examined in agoraphobic patients (Day et al., 2004).

Guided discovery helps the person to carefully evaluate the evidence for and against a troublesome belief. Sometimes a single question can be sufficient to bring about substantial cognitive and affective change, as the person contextualizes what seems like evidence for the belief among other autobiographical knowledge.

> PATIENT: I just know that I'm really stupid.
>
> THERAPIST: What makes you think that?
>
> PATIENT: My mother always said I had no common sense.
>
> THERAPIST: Was your mother some kind of expert on common sense?
>
> PATIENT: No! Everyone said she was a poor judge of character! (*Laughs.*)
>
> THERAPIST: So what does that say about your idea that you are really stupid?
>
> PATIENT: I guess I should examine it more closely. I think I have been giving her views too much weight—my husband always said she was ridiculously critical of me.

Here the patient's laughter suggests that the therapist's curiosity has evoked her own mental flexibility, so that she can bring other information to bear when she considers her mother's remarks. She can see them in a broader context, and an emotional shift has been achieved.

However, this process is usually more protracted, with much gathering and weighing of information. Detailed descriptions of the process of guided discovery can be found in various introductory books on cognitive therapy (J. S. Beck, 1995; Beck et al., 1979, 1985; Greenberger & Padesky, 1995; Leahy, 2003; Wells, 1997).

Where beliefs are entrenched a more elaborate technique can be used: the *historical test of schema*, in which the evidence for and against a particular belief can be carefully evaluated over a series of time periods in the patient's life (J. S. Beck, 1995; Padesky, 1994). Again, troublesome experiences are considered in a wider context.

> Polly had discovered that her adult daughter had been sexually assaulted as a child. She had developed PTSD following this revelation and felt very ashamed, as she had concluded that she must be a bad mother. After breaking her daughter's life down into periods of 2–5 years the patient was asked to review the evidence for and against this idea, while the therapist made notes. After studying the notes of this review the patient was happy to conclude that there was really no evidence for this harsh view of herself. The historical test of schema, combined with consideration of whether there were any signs that anything was wrong at the time of the abuse, led to a reduction in Polly's anxiety and shame.

Another excellent way to prompt for cognitive change is to use a range of *behavioral experiments*. In this process the patient is encouraged to formulate predictions about what might happen in a given situation. Clearly these predictions are largely based on thoughts, images, and memories arising from past experience. With the therapist's support the patient carefully observes what actually happens and then reflects on how this information relates to predictions arising from old beliefs and assumptions (for detailed discussion and many more examples see Chapter 6, and Bennett-Levy, Butler, et al., 2004).

> Rosa (see Chapter 2, p. 45) compared her image of spiders wanting to rush forward and bite her with what really happened when she visited the rather dusty apartment of a friend. She observed that far from dropping from the cobwebs and making a beeline for her the only spider in view took no notice of her, unlike the spiders in the film *Arachnophobia*.

Patients with social phobia often have images of themselves that are negative and distorted, and appear not have not been updated, following upsetting experiences of being bullied or criticized in their teens (Hackmann et al., 2000). To examine these images, and to help achieve some objective realism, it is useful to videotape a social interaction, then ask the patient to rate the way that he imagines he came across, and finally view and rate the video as objectively as possible, for the purpose of comparison (Harvey, Clark, Ehlers, & Rapee, 2000).

In agoraphobia, patients often have images of being humiliated or ignored in the event of a mental or physical catastrophe, resonating with earlier experiences of neglect, ridicule, or lack of protection (Day et al., 2004). Here one appropriate method of comparing image with reality is for the therapist to fake the feared catastrophe (e.g., fainting), so that the patient can observe whether the therapist is, for example, ignored, laughed at, or put in a straight jacket and locked up in hospital.

The importance of *comparing image against reality* is particularly marked in PTSD, where the patient can even enter a dissociative flashback and lose contact with present reality. In therapy, attempts are made to trigger the memories while helping the patient to stay grounded in the present, and discriminate between the "now" and the "then" (Ehlers et al., 2005).

> Susie had been attacked by a race horse she had looked after since it was born. She had perceived the horse as having turned into a monster just before it attacked her. She was terrified that anything even vaguely reminiscent of a horse could suddenly be transformed in this way, and could kill her. A picture of a horse in a friend's sitting room transported her back to the scene of the trauma, so that she experienced again the stable where it happened, and its characteristic smell. In the therapy session, pictures of foals and horses were projected onto a screen, and Susie was encouraged to gradually approach them. She was initially so scared that her legs gave way but gradually relaxed as she became aware that the pictures could not turn into real animals. Susie was helped in this process by being asked to describe everything about the experience that made it different from the trauma itself, for example, she was in an office, she was not alone, she was looking at a picture of a foal rather than being confronted by a real horse, and she was not in dan-

ger. This work was then extended by asking Susie to do more behavioral experiments to test whether anything reminiscent of a real horse might turn into a monster and kill her. This was tested using a series of small ornaments, toys, statues, and (eventually) real horses.

There is a range of ingenious experiments available to test metacognitive beliefs. For example, if a patient fears that having an image of someone experiencing an accident could actually make this happen the intrepid therapist can invite the patient to create images of accidents happening to the therapist, and see what (if anything) happens as a result (Bennett-Levy, Butler, et al., 2004).

When the belief to be challenged is a long-standing one that is hard to shift, the patient may be asked to use another schema change method: the *positive data log*. Every new experience that seems even weakly to support a new and positive belief or assumption (and disconfirm an old one) is carefully recorded and reflected upon in therapy, sometimes over a substantial period of time (J. S. Beck, 1995; Padesky, 1994).

Jack's father was very dominant and critical. As an adult Jack held the belief that he was useless. He began the slow process of keeping a written record of evidence that supported the new belief that he was seen by others as a worthwhile person. He made entries in a notebook of events that supported this belief and discussed them on a weekly basis with his therapist. Initially his entries were few and were given low ratings as supporting the new belief. However, his biased processing was gradually overcome, as he realized that in reality there was lots of evidence that he was indeed worthwhile.

USING THE PROPERTIES OF IMAGERY TO BRING ABOUT COGNITIVE CHANGE

Frequently the verbal and behavioral methods described above are woven together in skilful ways and bring about profound and lasting cognitive change. However, at times the patient may report that logic suggests that the original beliefs were distorted, but unfortunately this insight has not been accompanied by an emotional shift, and the fear persists. In such cases it may be helpful to turn to more experiential techniques, such as rescripting images, memories, or nightmares; working with metaphor; and so on (Arntz & Weertman, 1999; J. S. Beck, 2005; Edwards, 1989, 1990; Krakow, Kellner, Pathak, & Lambert, 1995; Krakow & Zadra, 2006; Young, Klosko, & Weishaar, 2003), often with good results. In this chapter we now provide a detailed examination of techniques utilizing imagery of various kinds. In the next chapter we intensify our focus on behavioral experiments, as another powerful method of bringing about whole-person change.

There are several aspects of imagery that make it likely to trigger maladaptive behavior. Images can be very convincing and are often incorrectly appraised as accurate reflections of past, present, or future reality. They can even be seen as real premonitions of disaster. People may believe that having the image in mind can affect the future, for better or worse. In addition, as we noted in Chapter 2, a person can experience upsetting images without being aware that there is input from memory, so that they signal a (misplaced) sense of current or future threat. Images and memories often appear to stop at the very worst point, not connecting to the fact that they could have (or did) end in a very different way.

Another complication is that memories can bleed into each other. Fragments of imagery, affect, and/or meaning related to a previous event can occur during another upsetting experience, creating a false impression of what happened during the more recent event. These appraisals can persist without being updated, as in the case of Karen, described in Chapter 2, page 44, who imagined her son struggling to breathe (like he did as a sickly infant) when removed from their burning house, whereas he had in fact been deeply unconscious at that point.

However the special properties of imagery can be utilized to bring about convincing shifts of perspective. The fact that images have face validity means that if a new and more realistic positive image can be evoked, this has some of the same potential as a good experience to bring about a shift in affect and beliefs. Imagery also seems to have some emergent properties: It often provides one with unexpected answers. Asking oneself questions such as "What is it about the image or memory that needs to be different for me to feel better about this?"; "What should have happened?"; or "What might be a more realistic way of seeing this?" often evokes a new, constructive perspective, incorporating more realistic metacognitive appraisals, and information about time code, the wider context, and ways in which the original contents were out of proportion (Wheatley, Brewin, Patel, & Hackmann, 2007).

Targeting Metacognitive Appraisals of Imagery

One method of changing the person's appraisals, so that she can see an image as simply a product of her own mind, is to demonstrate how one can play with an image and change it. For example, if a patient was asked to form an image of a giraffe and then suppress it, the image might well pop back, giving her the impression that the image could not be controlled. However, the therapist could suggest that the person could try to manipulate the image in some way: for example, imagining the giraffe bending his long neck to drink from a pool of water. This would demonstrate the malleability of imagery.

Moving on from this, there can sometimes be benefit in asking the patient to imagine that an upsetting image is framed, for example on a television screen, and that he is looking at it. This opens up the possibility of being able to switch it off, insert advertisements, smash the television, and so on, any of which might introduce an element of humor or playfulness, and convey the metacognitive message that this is only a product of his mind, and not necessarily something signaling a real threat.

> Jill was suffering from severe health anxiety and had become suicidal. She was lying in bed, crying almost incessantly, and could hardly sleep. She was refusing to see her child because she thought she would soon be dead, and her daughter should get used to her not being there. The therapist inquired about her thoughts and images, and the patient became even more agitated. She was picturing herself in a grave, with her husband and child visiting the graveyard with another woman her child called "mummy." Verbal challenging slightly weakened the idea that she would soon be dead, but the affect remained high.

The next step involved asking her to imagine that she was still alive and well, sitting on a sofa with her husband and daughter. She imagined that they were seeing the upsetting images on the TV screen and felt some relief when she imagined switching off the TV, smashing it and throwing it out of the window, and then driving off to see some friends. There was an intense emotional shift, following which she felt able to sleep again, see her daughter, and forget about the images. She had ceased to view them as premonitions.

This intervention had the effect of grounding the patient in the present, where she was still alive and well. In a similar way an imagery technique can be used to give a time code to an old memory and reduce the sense of current threat.

Barbara had been brutally sexually abused as a child, over a period of years. As an adult she was very anxious, and often suicidal. She had recurrent images of her erstwhile abuser coming to assault her again, even though she knew he was dead. To update this image and move it on the patient devised the following intervention: She imagined herself as she was in the present, flanked by two members of staff from the psychiatric hospital she attended. The abuser appeared and the patient spoke to him, telling him to go back into the past. She and the staff reminded him that he was dead now, and he could not hurt her anymore. She imagined him getting smaller and smaller, and further and further away, until he vanished. This gave her substantial relief.

Running the Image or Memory on Past the Worst Point

A simple but potentially powerful imagery intervention is to run the image on past the worst point. This provides the opportunity for the person to realize that even if something bad does (or did) happen there are possible rescue and coping factors that could be brought to bear, so that the dreaded event might have a beginning, a middle, and a (possibly positive) end.

John had become afraid of vomiting in public, following a humiliating experience when he got drunk while out with friends, and they mocked him. He was invited to dinner with his brother and his new wife but had a disturbing image of being sick as soon as he arrived. The therapist asked him to visualize this "worst case scenario," but to run the image on past the worst point. John did so and imagined that he was sick, but his brother was sympathetic. He and his wife cleaned up quickly, by which time John was feeling much better, and was able to enjoy the evening.

During reliving of traumatic memories the process of running on past the worst moments may help the fear reduce, as connections are made between what the person feared and what really happened.

During a serious accident a patient had an image of her legs being shattered and the bones sticking out. However, only a moment later she looked down and realized she was not nearly as badly hurt as she had feared. Running on past the worst point of this hot spot helped diminish the associated emotion.

Such an intervention can surprisingly often be reassuring to the patient. However, in some cases it has the opposite effect. For some people, it fleshes out further drastic aspects of the anxiety equation, and the image runs on in a way that illustrates the likely interpersonal consequences of the feared catastrophe, and the person's perceived inability to cope with them. In such a case the intervention provides more information for the conceptualization, but other strategies will need to be utilized to bring about change.

Placing Fragments of Memory in a Broader Context

As described in Chapter 2 fragments of upsetting memories can carry distorted meanings that have not been updated. Guided discovery and behavioral experiments can be used to challenge these appraisals. Frequently the patient will remark that logically she can see that her appraisals were distorted, but this does not necessarily change the associated affect. Several procedures may be used to help bring emotions into line with the new appraisals.

At the simplest level a memory can be updated by asking the patient to relive it in the first person, present tense, and following each "hot spot" with its distorted meaning by asking "And what do you know about that now?" The answers may come spontaneously, or may have previously been arrived at during guided discovery, while drawing out what happened, or via behavioral experiments (Ehlers & Clark, 2000; Grey et al., 2002). As the narrative begins to develop into a more realistic account the patient may be asked to write out the new version of events, highlighting any updating (Ehlers, Hackmann, & Michael, 2004). This process can be utilized in PTSD, but also in other anxiety disorders where there are intrusive memories carrying distorted meanings.

If this does not shift belief ratings or decrease upsetting affect, imagery can be used to help a patient place an upsetting fragment of memory with a distorted or overgeneralized meaning into a broader, less toxic context, and thus change the meaning.

Roberta was suffering from social phobia and was convinced that others would not like her. She described how she felt in social situations by saying that she felt as if there was a banner over her head with the words "show-off" emblazoned on it. This was the way that her mother had described her in public when she was small, on a number of humiliating occasions. Verbal discussion suggested that her mother had favored her sister, who suffered from ill health, and that other people did not share her mother's harsh view of Roberta. She finally arrived at an imagery scenario in which she visited a wizard who had a crystal ball. In the crystal ball, scenes from her childhood could be clearly seen. Roberta watched the pictures change until finally she saw herself filling a hot-water bottle for her mother, something she did every night. Over this final picture another banner appeared, bearing the word "kind." Roberta cried as she realized that her mother's criticism had given her too harsh a view of herself.

Peter was involved in a car crash. Some nurses passed by, and Peter felt sure they would stop and help him. However, they just walked straight past the car. This plunged Peter into a familiar sense of abandonment and neglect. His needs had often been ignored when he was a child. His appraisal was that no one cared about him, even though he knew that only a moment later several other people had come to his assistance. To shift the felt sense the therapist suggested that he viewed the accident from another perspective: Peter imagined himself viewing it from above and realized that as the nurses walked past other people were running forward to help him. He concluded that the nurses would have been able to see them too, and might have felt that they could safely leave his care to them. This transformation of the image brought emotion into line with logic, and Peter felt less bleak about the incident.

Transforming Childhood Memories

Quite similar processes can be used to change the meanings carried by disturbing childhood memories. Imagery techniques are utilized by a number of cognitive therapists working with Axis II disorders. These may be described as experiential techniques, though the aim is to bring about cognitive change (Arntz & Weertman, 1999; Hackmann, 2005a; Smucker, Dancu, Foa, & Niederee, 1995; Weertman & Arntz, 2007; Wild et al., 2007; Young et al., 2003). For example, Arntz and Weertman (1999) described a process that involves identifying a childhood memory laden with negative schematic meaning, asking the patient to relive the memory from the child's perspective; then relive it from the perspective of the patient's adult self who sees what is happening and may intervene; and finally relive it again from the perspective of the child (who sees the reactions of the adult self) and is asked what else the patient would like to happen. This process involves asking the patient to imagine things that never really happened. Also in severe cases the patient may be asked to only relive a small part of the traumatic experience before proceeding to the rescripting phase. The rationale is not an exposure or habituation rationale but focuses instead on changing affect and appraisals.

However, the procedure can have powerful effects, and results of a randomized controlled trial suggest that in personality disorder restructuring early memories can be as effective as other more analytic schema change methods (Weertman & Arntz, 2007). Our clinical experience suggests that (when effective) the result of this work is that beliefs change to more realistic, measured appraisals than those made at the time, and affect drops. In this process memories have been accessed, reflected upon, and put in a broader context. If the intervention is effective the event is seen as an isolated event (or string of events) in the past: an exception rather than the basis for a rule about how the self and others are perceived. In short, some cognitive-emotional processing has occurred.

Cognitive therapists vary in the extent to which such techniques are given a cognitive rationale. It remains an empirical question as to whether the effects of experiential techniques would be enhanced or diminished by more thoroughly interweaving them with our more traditional cognitive techniques and embedding the imagery work among guided discovery and behavioral experiments. Such an approach was suggested some years ago (Edwards, 1990). Preliminary results suggest that significant effects of this technique can be produced in social phobia, after a single session in which verbal discussion and memory restructuring are interwoven (Wild et al., 2007). The steps in this procedure are described together with a worked example in Figure 5.1. In this figure an approach is suggested in which verbal discussion plays a part in deciding how to modify the imagery. However, this is sometimes omitted, and the imagery transformation simply arises in response to guided consideration of possible changes, prompted by the use of questions such as "What would need to happen to make you feel better about this? Can you imagine that actually happening?"

Summary

To summarize, the basic principles outlined above suggest that the following procedures can be used in varying combinations to bring about cognitive-emotional processing:

1. Evoke the hot material, that is, thoughts, images, memories, and so on (some spontaneous change occurs).
2. Prompt for further cognitive change.
3. Use the special properties of imagery to bring about or strengthen belief and affect shifts.

Specific techniques can be selected to:

1. Change metacognitive appraisals, by manipulating or framing an image.
2. Add a time code, lessen the sense of current threat.
3. Run on past the worst point.
4. See things from a different perspective.
5. Update memory, place fragments of memory or imagery in a broader context among other memories or new information.

These same principles and similar procedures can also be used to work with more metaphorical imagery and dreams or nightmares.

UNPACKING AND TRANSFORMING METAPHORICAL IMAGES

Accessing and Unpacking Metaphors and Metaphorical Images in Cognitive Therapy

Collaboration and case formulation can be improved by paying attention to the metaphors used by patients, and making summaries using their own words. This also allows for elaboration of new perspectives and ways of dealing with potential obstacles.

Ray was beginning to recover after several traumatic experiences and was making some tentative plans for the future. The therapist used the metaphor of things beginning to sprout in a garden. However, the patient spoke of building founda-

Identifying a significant memory

The patient may describe an intrusive, upsetting memory, or a memory may be identified by using the emotional bridge technique (p. 42), starting with a recurrent image or felt sense. Select a memory that carries meanings that still color experience in the present.

A patient with social phobia had a recurrent image of herself with big ears, feeling as if she was about to be confronted by bullies. Linked this to experiences of being bullied by friends, in her teens. Had an upsetting memory of going to a party where she knew hardly anyone, and hearing her friend shouting that if she was the girl with the big ears she was not welcome.

Reliving the memory

The memory is relived (as in PTSD) in the first person, present tense, with a great deal of detail about thoughts and feelings (usually done with closed eyes).

The patient relived the memory and reported feeling very anxious and embarrassed. She could see herself with big ears (from the observer perspective), alone but about to face the bullies.

Identifying the meanings given to this event, and taking belief ratings

The therapist asks the patient what this memory means about the self, others, and the world; takes belief ratings; asks about the emotions aroused; and asks for affect ratings.

The patient explained that she believed that she was ugly and unacceptable (100%), that others would be hostile and rejecting (90%), and that she had no backup (100%).

Checking that these meanings still persist today

The therapist checks that these are still troublesome beliefs the patient holds today.

She reported that this was how she felt in public, in the present.

Evaluating evidence for and against the appraisals made at the time of the event

Guided discovery is used to search for additional information and alternative perspectives.

Through a process of guided discovery the patient reflected on the nature of the friendship. She had been close to these girls until they got heavily involved with drugs and wanted her to join them. When she refused, they rejected and bullied her. This left her feeling humiliated and alone. However, when she considered their lives in the present she realized that they had ended up being viewed as losers. Neither had a job, or a steady boyfriend. On the other hand, she was about to get married and had a job she enjoyed. She still lived in the same town and knew that these girls were not well regarded, even by their own families.

Reliving the memory and prompting for updating by asking questions*

The patient relives the memory including appraisals made at the time, and therapist inquires what the patient knows now that might lead to another conclusion.

This step was omitted.

(continued)

FIGURE 5.1. Worked example: Transforming the meaning of a memory.

Transforming the memory by inserting imaginal material more in accord with realistic appraisals

If the beliefs and affect have not dropped significantly the patient can experiment with an imagery transformation. Several attempts may be made to arrive at a more realistic perspective.

The patient rescripted the memory by imagining that she was meeting her friends again, as an adult. This time she saw the scene as if through her own eyes, and faced the bullies head-on. She was not aware of her ears. She imagined lots of friends and family coming, as well as relations of the bullies. She imagined each person choosing who he or she would back in this situation, until the patient had a real sense of just how much back-up she had in the present, while her old friends were alone, and were now seen as the "losers."

Checking the belief and affect ratings

The therapist checks the ratings to ensure that a new perspective has been reached.

The beliefs had shifted to 10% ugly or unacceptable, 20% others will be hostile, and 0% I have no back-up. Significant changes in mood and behavior followed.

---

*Not every step is included every time. See text.

FIGURE 5.1. *(continued)*

tions and making steps, metaphors he returned to the following week. The therapist reflected his use of language, leading the patient to explain that in a sense he was building his own castle, carefully but well. As he climbed the steps he was aware of strong rubber bands that could pull him back down. These were the assumptions of his family, which had proved to be more of a hindrance than a help, and which he needed to cut through carefully as he progressed up the stairs, to avoid a possible relapse. These assumptions were then identified and modified, and finally the modified versions were included in his relapse prevention package (see Chapter 10).

It is also possible to access meanings being given to difficult situations by considering metaphorical images that arise on prompting after dwelling on a specific, recent occurrence and how it made the patient feel. This can then be "unpacked" as described in Chapter 2, to uncover the appraisals underpinning the distress. Once the patient is fully in touch with the implicational level of meaning given to the event she can stay with the imagery, reflecting on what would need to be different in the image for her to feel better about the situation, and what shift there might need to be in her assumptions or behavior to bring this about (Edwards, 1989). An example is given in Figure 5.2. This incorporates sections in which the patient is invited as part of the process to put meanings into words at different points, linking the work to the formulation, and exploring old and new assumptions and core beliefs. Some therapists may delay direct discussion of meaning until the end of the exercise.

In Figure 5.3 a similar exercise is presented, using drawing as a method of producing images that can be reflected upon in cognitive therapy (Johles, 2005). The pauses for relaxation and positive imagery can be omitted, although there is some evidence that relaxation permits the emergence of more vivid imagery, and also places the disturbing

Exploring the "felt sense"

Focus on a recurrent problem, a typical upsetting situation. Bring to mind a recent example, focusing on the emotions felt in that situation. Reflect on thoughts and feelings, and exactly what is experienced in the body.

The patient reported feeling oppressed by her demanding mother. She was aware of tension and stiffness in her back.

Evoking a metaphor

Having tuned in to the whole "felt sense," let a metaphorical image arise that somehow stands for how all this feels. When an image arises try to stay with it, even if seems odd or banal. If several occur, choose the one that seems to be the most compelling.

The patient reported that she felt as if she had an old-fashioned washboard on her back.

Exploring the metaphor

Consider all the sensory aspects of the image: sights, sounds, smells, size, texture, and so on. Also what it looks like from various angles, and distances, and associated feelings.

On closer examination of the image, she exclaimed that the washboard was becoming ingrown, and embedded in her skin. This felt threatening. In addition, her mother was hiding behind her back, and her hands were like claws, reaching out for something.

Reflecting on the meaning*

Reflect on the meaning of this metaphorical image for the problem: What does it mean about the self, about others, and about the world? What is the history of this image? Does it resonate with any past experiences?

The image suggested to the patient that her mother was treating her like a domestic servant, but in rather a manipulative, sneaky way. The washboard was linked to memories of a domestic help her mother had employed in Africa when she was young, to wash their clothes by hand. It felt as if this pattern of relationship could be bad for her health.

Considering change

If this metaphor represents a predicament what needs to happen to resolve the problem? What would need to change within the image? What would need to happen in real life?

The patient felt that the problem in their relationship needed to be acknowledged, and some consideration needed to be given to ways in which her mother's needs could be met without taking such a toll on the patient.

Visualizing change

Staying with the metaphorical image, try to see these changes taking place and find ways of changing the picture to make this happen. May need to try a number of changes before a worthwhile shift occurs. Some changes that seem easy in prospect may prove impossible. There will be a change in affect, and the change will feel steady and complete, when the shift of perspective is made.

(continued)

FIGURE 5.2. Exploring and transforming a metaphorical image: Instructions and worked example.

The patient considered how to have the washboard removed from her back. Surgery seemed inappropriate. What needed to happen was that the washboard had to float out of her back. When she visualized this it appeared that the washboard was still attached to her by a rope round her neck. She needed help to deal with this: She visualized her husband removing the washboard by cutting the rope. Next, she imagined the three of them considering the washboard as it sat in front of them, and making proper plans for the care her mother needed.

Reflecting on the new metaphorical image and its meaning*

If it feels better like this, what does the new metaphor mean, about the self, others, and the world? If it were possible to see the situation like this how would this change the emotions and other reactions?

From this the patient concluded that the pattern of this relationship needed to change. She would need to be more direct and assertive with her mother and would need the moral support of her husband to try some problem solving to decide what would be the best way to help her, without getting worn out herself. This called into question her old assumption, that she should always put the needs of others first.

Planning to test the new perspective*

In what situations could the new perspective be tested out? How could this be achieved (i.e., what would be appropriate behavioral experiments)?

The patient decided she would share her concerns with her husband and suggested that together they would approach her mother. They could then embark on a constructive discussion with her about what to do next. She did this and was pleasantly surprised at her mother's reasonable response.

---

*Elements of reflection on meaning, verbal challenging, and behavioral experiments may be interwoven with imagery in cognitive therapy.

FIGURE 5.2. *(continued)*

material in a broader context by bringing to awareness the fact that safe and happy places exist.

Rescripting Nightmares

Similar principles can be used to restructure mental representations arising in dreams and nightmares. There is a saying that "A nightmare is a dream you have not had the courage to end," and it is true that in a nightmare the person often wakes at the very worst moment, for example, during recurring nightmares following trauma. A number of studies report beneficial effects from desensitization (e.g., Cellucci & Lawrence, 1978), and good results have also been obtained by running through the nightmare and giving it a different ending, or changing significant elements in the dream to make it less distressing (see Krakow et al., 1995; Krakow & Zadra, 2006; Marks, 1978). A 70% reduction in nightmares has been reported after only one imagery rehearsal session, followed by self-practice (Kellner, Neidhardt, Krakow, & Pathak, 1992). In Krakow's studies transforming the content of nightmares using imagery rehearsal brought about a drop in the frequency and severity of nightmares in PTSD, and a simultaneous drop in other PTSD symptoms including intrusive memories.

The exercise can start with a period of relaxation,* perhaps accompanied by an image of a peaceful place to which the patient can return between each of the imagery and drawing steps. The therapist then poses a series of questions:

"How is your life at the moment?"

The patient lets a metaphorical image arise, then draws a picture.

Relaxation and positive imagery*

"What is your next step: what is emerging for you?"

The patient lets a metaphorical image arise, then draws it.

Relaxation and positive imagery*

"What barriers or obstacles are there?"

The patient lets a metaphorical image arise, then draws it.

Relaxation and positive imagery*

"What qualities do you need to help you deal with these?"

The patient lets a metaphorical image arise, then draws it.

Relaxation and positive imagery*

The therapist then encourages the patient to reflect on what the pictures convey, about the patient's view of the situation, and what it means about the self, world, and others, and old and new beliefs and assumptions that could be tested against reality.

----

*Periods of relaxation and positive imagery can be omitted. See text.

FIGURE 5.3. A drawing exercise as described by Johles (2005).

Conversely, reliving and restructuring traumatic memories using the methods described above can lead to a steady reduction not only in intrusive daytime memories but also in nightmares, as well an improved quality of sleep (Hackmann, 2005b). This supports the idea that intrusive memories and nightmares are signs of incomplete emotional processing, which can be resolved by restructuring the imagery. Possible processes involved include the realization that both are only products of the mind (see Chapter 4) and therefore amenable to change; placing the traumatic material in a broader context, so that it can be seen as only part of the story; and giving it a time code and updating the content so that it can be seen as input from memory rather than having current significance.

Once again this work does not always have to be embedded among other cognitive techniques but seems to be effective in its own right, as in the studies mentioned above. However, this poses another empirical question: Would the effectiveness of this procedure be enhanced by reflecting on the meaning and history of the dreams or nightmares, and the possible cognitive distortions that are apparent, and available for potential transformation? This is a topic that was explored by Beck and colleagues in the early days of cognitive therapy but has still not been thoroughly researched in the anxiety disorders (Beck & Hurvich, 1959; Beck & Ward, 1961; Freeman, 1981). Figure 5.4 provides an example of a possible way of working with a nightmare within a cognitive framework. This patient's treatment and history were summarized at the end of Chapter 1.

CONCLUSION

In this chapter we described a variety of methods of not only bringing about cognitive change but also facilitating full emotional processing, within the framework of cognitive therapy. We have given a full account of strategies that address intrusive material, carrying meanings that are out of context, out of proportion, or with an incorrect time code. The methods involve various combinations of evoking the hot material, reflecting upon it, and assembling more information in a way that transforms the old, distorted meanings. Techniques involving imagery and memories were described in greater detail, as they are perhaps less widely used yet often go beyond verbal methods in bringing about lasting, whole-person change. They can also be dovetailed with behavioral experiments, another powerful experiential technique, described in full in the next chapter.

Evoking a description of a nightmare

The patient is asked to describe the recurrent nightmare in the first person, present tense, and to reflect on its meaning.

The patient describes the nightmare, in which he is a tiny person in a huge car or ball, moving at great speed. He cannot reach the controls and feels absolutely powerless (therapeutic interventions and history summarized at the close of Chapter 1).

Reflection on meaning, and history of the elements in the nightmare*

This is the point to consider the meanings encapsulated in the nightmare, and possible cognitive distortions.

This is how he felt during the traffic accident. His vehicle was knocked sideways, and he had a struggle to keep it upright, and manage to drive it off the road. When he came to a halt he could not remember if he had hit any other cars and feared that he had left a trail of carnage. He is left with a fear of losing control of the car while driving.
The work he has done in therapy has helped him fill in the gaps in his understanding. He now knows that he did manage to control the vehicle, and get it off the road without causing any damage. He was always a good driver, and the accident was not his fault. The feeling of being tiny and having no control on the road is colored by memories of being physically abused by his stepbrothers, as a tiny child, but he is now a grown man.

Reflection on how to change the nightmare*

The patient is asked to reflect on what elements of the nightmare he would like to change, to make the nightmare less distressing, and *(when using cognitive therapy) to bring it in line with a more realistic appraisal of what happened in the past, or is likely to happen in the future.

The patient decides that he needs first to imagine that he is driving, feeling as if he is tiny, the road is vast, and he has no control of the car. Then he needs to switch to the realization that this is only an illusion, and in reality he is a big man, fully able to reach the controls. Finally he decides to finish the nightmare scenario by imagining that he is driving confidently down the main road, then turning off, and parking the car.

Evoking the nightmare again, imagining the selected changes in the scenario

The patient describes himself sitting in the car, feeling tiny and out of control. Then he lets himself become aware of his broad shoulders and long legs. He feels quietly confident and drives happily along the road. He can easily reach the controls and skillfully negotiates his passage through the heavy traffic. He turns off the main road and parks the car before locking up and walking off.

Homework

The patient was asked to practice this imaginary scenario at home, and advised that if he woke with the nightmare he could carry it on past the worst point, and transform the ending in this more realistic manner.

---

*This description involves direct reflection on meaning, and some verbal challenging. See text.

FIGURE 5.4. Rescripting a nightmare: Instructions and worked example.

SIX

The Role of Behavioral Experiments

In cognitive therapy, our prime objective is to achieve congruent cognitive, behavioral, and (perhaps most important) emotional change. As we indicated in our introduction to this section of the book, our aim as therapists is not to give patients an intellectual appreciation of the role of cognition in emotional distress, and how in theory cognitions might be modified. Rather we hope to facilitate a profound transformation, not only in what patients think, but also in what they feel and what they do. Chapter 5 described how working with images, metaphors, and memories can enhance this process. In this chapter we turn to another powerful means of enhancing whole-person transformation: experiential learning through behavioral experiments.

Experiments encourage learning on many levels (see Bennett-Levy, Butler, et al., 2004). At the most fundamental level, they offer opportunities for the formation of new stimulus–response associations. Reflection on experience promotes declarative knowledge (knowing that . . .), while planning and experience support the acquisition of procedural knowledge (knowing how to . . . , "riding a bike" knowledge). A robust finding in the literature on memory is that actions that we perform ourselves are better remembered than actions we only observe or hear about ("the enactment effect"; Engelkamp, 1998). Engelkamp (1998) suggested that this may be because "during enactment a rich awareness of the learning episode develops"; that is, multimodal processing occurs, including not only verbal and conceptual elements, but also visual, sensory, and motor elements. Enactive methods like behavioral experiments engage the whole person in the learning process (thinking, emotion, physiology, behavior), resulting in multisensory, emotionally charged, self-referent memories that are deeply processed and so more likely to be recalled. Behavioral experiments, when well designed and attentively debriefed, can provide patients with "experience—something that can be incorporated into the stuff of my identity, that can be felt in the bones" (Hoffman, 1989, p. 194). Thus direct experience of behaving in new ways, especially in a real-life context, increases the chances of "gut-level learning"—rational and emotional mind changing together, head and heart in concert (Epstein, 1998).

In this chapter, we consider the value to patients of direct experiential learning and offer practical guidelines for conducting effective behavioral experiments. To illustrate the process, we describe in some detail a particular case, whose story follows.

Illustrative Case Example: The Story of Alan

Alan grew up as an only child on a farm on the outskirts of a small village. His father was withdrawn and irritable, and his mother frequently preoccupied. There was little or no affection, physical contact, or warmth. At the age of 5, Alan began attending the village school. He was a quiet, shy child and quickly became a target for teasing and bullying by peers. They told him that he was "a psycho" and "weird." None of the teachers protected or helped him, though he had the sense that they knew what was happening. Anxiety made him academically slow, and that too became a focus for bullying and shame. Alan was the last in his year to enter puberty. This provided his peers with more ammunition for ridicule.

By the time he left school, Alan had concluded that other people were "out to get him" and avoided them whenever he could. He saw himself as odd and different—in fact monstrous, barely human. He felt uptight and self-conscious whenever he had to be around people, and protected himself as best he could by lurking in the background, refusing eye contact, hunching down so as to make himself insignificant, and responding aggressively if he thought someone was about to attack (this sometimes triggered answering aggression from others, who were unable to see the intense sense of vulnerability behind it). He managed to find work with his hands, which suited him, and had one or two acquaintances he could talk to in the pub. But he lived alone, never dared to seek relationships with women and, as he entered his mid-30s, felt increasingly sad and lonely—life was passing him by. At times, he became so depressed and hopeless that killing himself seemed the only solution. Once his mood dipped, his drive to engage with life reduced even further, and he would spend days shut up in his room, brooding and feeling increasing despair.

Alan realized that his experiences had damaged his sense of himself, and that his life was painfully constricted by fear. He first sought help by asking his family doctor for medication. This had some impact on the physical signs of anxiety, but it did not lead to any fundamental change in how he saw himself or led his life. He then turned to counseling and found that it helped him for the first time to appreciate why he saw things as he did, and to begin to feel that perhaps everything was not his fault. But increased understanding once again did not lead to any real change.

Alan then found out about cognitive therapy through the Internet and contacted a local center. His goals were clear: He didn't want to spend more time talking about things and delving into the past, he wanted to change how he felt about himself and other people, to start living with more freedom and confidence, and to open up the long-term possibility of finding a wife and establishing a family of his own. Although the prospect terrified him, he recognized that he would have to take the risk of doing things differently if he was to have any chance of achieving what he wanted.

THE ROLE OF BEHAVIOR IN MAINTAINING ANXIETY

The role of avoidance of feared stimuli in perpetuating anxiety has been noted since behavioral principles and procedures were initially developed in the first half of the 20th century. There is an intuitive logic to avoidance: If something is frightening, then it makes sense to keep away from it and, if that is not possible, to escape from it as soon as possible. Behavioral and cognitive therapies acknowledge that avoidance and escape keep anxiety in place. From a classical behavioral perspective, they prevent extinction or habituation of learned fear responses. From a cognitive perspective, they prevent old ideas from being updated in the light of experience. Either way, the main clinical implication is that, if you wish to overcome anxiety, there is no alternative but to face the situations you fear.

However, simple avoidance and escape are only part of the picture. A more recent development highlights the importance of what people deliberately do or do not do (as they see it) to prevent anticipated bad things from happening. Salkovskis's (1991) concept of "safety-seeking behaviors" has helped us to understand a conundrum central to anxiety: how people can repeatedly experience feared situations in which the worst does *not* happen, and yet their anxiety continues without meaningful change. Safety-seeking behaviors are the reason for this: They are the precautions people take to prevent their fears from coming true. In the immediate term, such precautions help the person to feel more secure, in that they give the impression that harm has successfully been averted ("If I had not done that, then . . ."). In the longer term, they contribute to problem maintenance because they make it impossible to test the accuracy of unhelpful cognitions. Indeed, they may unwittingly make the problem worse. So, for example, Alan's sharply aggressive response when he feared attack alienated people who might in fact have been benignly disposed toward him (and indeed had an impact on the therapeutic relationship, in that his therapist sometimes felt she was being cut down to size and treated with contempt). Again, the implication is that anxiety will continue unless feared situations are faced. But unless at the same time safety-seeking behaviors are abandoned, then the sense of danger barely averted will persist, and patients will continue to believe that if they had *not* taken precautions, the harm they anticipated would indeed have occurred.

A range of behaviors may be disrupted by anxiety, and it can have a broad impact on people's lives. This is especially true when the anxiety is not straightforward but is rooted in highly aversive early experiences and comorbid with other difficulties such as depression, hopelessness, and low self-esteem. Alan's case illustrates this. Not only were his opportunities for social contact and intimacy restricted by anxious concerns, but his academic achievement had suffered, with a resulting constriction in the career opportunities open to him. His leisure activities too were constrained by anxiety: Most of his activities were solitary. Even the extent to which he looked after himself was compromised. He tended to rush while shopping so as to avoid human contact, grabbing food randomly instead of ensuring that he ate a nourishing and balanced diet. He would have liked to go to a local gym but was afraid it would involve talking to people. Awareness of these restrictions and hopelessness about the possibility of change triggered depression, which further reduced his energy and motivation to do anything that might extend his range.

BEHAVIORAL INTERVENTIONS IN TREATMENT

Cognitive therapists frequently endorse the value of behavioral interventions in establishing new perspectives and giving them gut-level credibility. Clark (1989), for example, noted that behavioral interventions "can be one of the most effective ways of changing beliefs" (p. 82). That said, the concept of the schema (e.g., Clark & Beck, 1999; Teasdale & Barnard, 1993) suggests that to focus exclusively on any one aspect of functioning is to oversimplify. Recurrent response patterns are neither exclusively cognitive nor exclusively behavioral—or indeed exclusively affective or physiological. Rather they can rather be understood as constellations of interlinked elements, which may not be entirely synchronous (Hodgson & Rachman, 1974) but which, broadly speaking, covary over time. Thus triggering one element of the system will tend to trigger other associated elements. In anxiety, for example, a sense that something bad is about to happen (cognition) will tend to be accompanied by a subjective feeling of anxiety or dread (emotion), by signs of arousal (physiology), and by attempts to take evasive action or engage in self-protective maneuvers (behavior). These ideas have clear practical implications: In treating anxiety, we should aim not just for cognitive change, but for change across the system as a whole—cognitive, emotional, physical, and behavioral. Clinical experience illustrates the effects of failing to achieve this. For example, patients whose behavior has changed may nonetheless still feel they have good reason to be anxious, whereas others remark at the end of a cognitive intervention: "I see what you *mean*, but I still *feel* the same." In addressing these common problems in cognitive therapy, behavioral experiments play a crucial role.

Bennett-Levy, Westbrook, and colleagues (2004) defined behavioral experiments as follows:

> Behavioral experiments are planned experiential activities, based on experimentation or observation, which are undertaken by patients in or between cognitive therapy sessions. Their design is derived directly from a cognitive formulation of the problem, and their primary purpose is to obtain new information which may help to:
>
> - Test the validity of the patients' existing beliefs about themselves, others, and the world.
> - Construct and/or test new, more adaptive beliefs.
> - Contribute to the development and verification of the cognitive formulation. (p. 8)

An example of the first of these was a sequence of experiments Alan carried out to test his prediction that people would attack him if he approached them (described in more detail below). An example of the second occurred when this sequence of experiments suggested that his predictions were not in fact correct. On the basis of these results, he tentatively formulated a new expectation ("Most people are OK and can be approached safely"), and began to operate from it, and to observe the results. An example of the third was when, at the very beginning of therapy, it was not entirely clear what cognitions accounted for the intensity of his fear of others. To help make sense of this, the therapist (with his agreement) arranged for him to have a short conversation with a work colleague. Inquiring into his reactions before, during, and after the conversation clarified what ran through his mind when he encountered others. That is, he predicted that the work colleague would instantly judge him as somehow monstrous and treat him with hostility and contempt. He had difficulty knowing how she did in fact respond, because his attention was captured by his own state of anxiety, and because he avoided looking at her and did everything to cut the encounter short. These safety-seeking behaviors made the colleague wonder what she had done to offend him. Finally, he would brood on the encounter, seeking out signs of rejection (e.g., the colleague's evident awkwardness with him was interpreted as a sign that his predictions were true, rather than as a consequence of his own self-protective maneuvers). These findings, together with information from the initial assessment session, were summarized in a relatively simply formulation diagram (Figure 6.1).

We now outline how to plan, carry out, and evaluate behavioral experiments successfully, so that they provide patients with opportunities for effective experiential learning. We pay particular attention to the value of therapist-guided, in-session experiments and highlight some of the difficulties that can arise in less-than-straightforward cases.

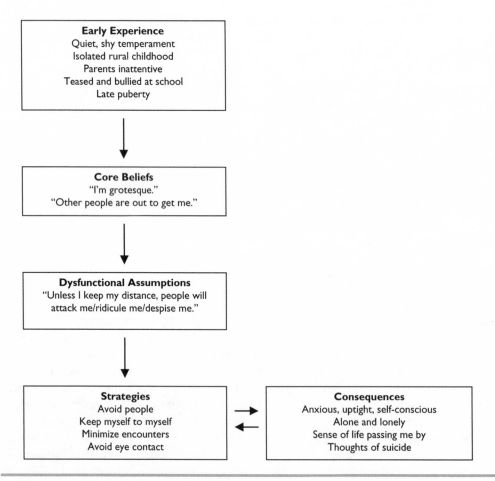

FIGURE 6.1. Alan's initial case formulation.

BEHAVIORAL EXPERIMENTS AND EXPERIENTIAL LEARNING

We have proposed elsewhere (Bennett-Levy, Butler, et al., 2004) that an illuminating framework for understanding and using behavioral experiments can be found in ideas derived, not from psychotherapy, but from adult learning theory and education. These propose that learning in adults is fostered by the creation of a learning culture that in many ways mirrors the style of cognitive therapy ("androgogy"; Knowles, 1990; Knowles, Holton, & Swanson, 2005). Knowles advocated an essentially collaborative learning framework, in which the educator has a facilitative (rather than didactic) role, encouraging experiential learning, independent inquiry, questioning, and curiosity. The learner adopts a complementary stance: independent, self-reliant, and active. This seems entirely consistent with what is expected of patients in classical short-term cognitive therapy for specific disorders, but for more complex cases with high comorbidity and personality issues, attaining this self-initiating stance might be a gradual process over the whole course of therapy.

In adult learning as conceived by Knowles, the learner's experience is valued, and indeed used as a resource in the learning process (this echoes the respectful stance of cognitive therapy toward the patient's expertise in his or her own life). The structure of learning, rather than being predetermined by a rigid syllabus, is flexibly responsive to the problems, questions, and needs of the learner. Interestingly, though this stance would be routine in ordinary clinical practice, flexibility and responsiveness to the individual can be real challenges for the model-based treatment protocols for specific disorders that we described earlier, especially when delivered within a research context that requires consistency of approach across all participants. In adult learning, ideally, the motivation for learning is intrinsic: curiosity, the pleasure of acquiring knowledge and practicing new skills, personal growth. In the case of cognitive therapy for anxiety, perhaps, we might hope for a genuine desire to move forward, to reduce stress and anxiety, to find personally relevant solutions to problems, to improve the quality of life, and increase well-being and self-confidence (rather than, e.g., "My doctor said I should come").

The Learning Process in Cognitive Therapy

Knowles's ideas provide a broad framework for characterizing the nature of the learning culture within cognitive therapy. Kolb's (1984) "learning circle," designed to map the process of experiential learning in adults in greater detail, suggests that for effective learning and retention to occur, learners must follow through a sequence of steps: experience, observation, reflection, and planning (Bennett-Levy, Butler, et al., 2004, Chapters 1 and 2; see Figure 6.2).

"Experience" refers to direct action or experience—doing something. In the context of this chapter, "experience" refers in particular to the behavioral experiment itself—approaching where avoidance has been habitual, dropping safety-seeking behaviors, risking behaving in new ways where the outcome is uncertain, and so on.

"Observation" means paying careful attention to the nature of experience (see Chapter 5)—mindful awareness, to borrow from another conceptual framework. Observation is purely descriptive, not analytical. Initially, it may be done only retrospectively, especially if people are caught up at the time in the drama of their own distress-

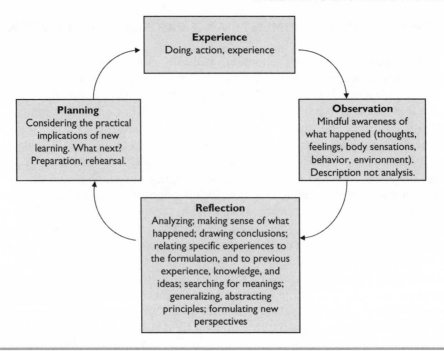

FIGURE 6.2. Kolb's learning circle.

ing thoughts and emotions and are unable to decenter from what is going on. In cognitive therapy, for example, sessions regularly include reviewing exactly what happened during upsetting events that have occurred since patient and therapist last met: what situation triggered the distress; what thoughts, emotions, and body sensations were present; what the person did; what the person noticed happening around him or her; and so forth. With practice these various aspects of experience can be captured as they actually occur, so that observation is present alongside experience.

"Reflection" means making sense of the experience (analysis, assigning meaning). At this stage the patient is relating his or her observations to prior knowledge (including the conceptualization), checking out what actually happened against his or her expectations, considering whether what has been observed validates or contradicts higher order assumptions or beliefs, and so forth. This is also where new knowledge is put into words (made declarative), where general principles of change are derived from specific experiences (e.g., "Take it in small steps"), and overarching metamessages abstracted (e.g., "Just because I think something, it doesn't mean it's true"). Thus reflection facilitates the ongoing process of relating the specific to the general, and the general to the specific. This two-way traffic increases the chances that learning in particular situations will affect higher order beliefs, and that work on higher order beliefs will be firmly rooted in day-to-day changes in thinking and behavior (the sandwich principle, Chapter 3, p. 64).

"Planning," finally, refers to thinking ahead, working out what the practical implications of new understanding might be, what predictions now need to be tested, how this might be done, what new discoveries need to be made, and where to go next. Thus planning forms a foundation for the next experience (experiment). This tells us that the term "learning circle" is in a sense a misnomer—the sequence in fact describes a continuing process, in which each cycle leads naturally to the beginning of another, and so to further learning. Over a course of therapy, therefore, patients may complete the circle many times, sometimes consolidating existing learning through repetition of a successful outcome, sometimes investigating and gathering data, sometimes using one completed circle as a basis for taking another new step.

Experiential learning frameworks like Kolb's suggest that experience alone and of itself (doing stuff) does not produce change, and they do so in terms that cognitive therapists will readily recognize: "When we undergo an experience, this does not always lead to new insights and new learning. For example, if the experience only serves to confirm already held beliefs it will be interpreted as supporting the existing cognitive status quo and little attention will be paid to it. . . . We have to engage with the experience and reflect on what happened, how it happened and why" (Beard & Wilson, 2002, p. 17). In fact, aspects of cognitive therapy can facilitate each element of the learning circle. For example, the development of observation skills is encouraged by self-monitoring (including the first three columns of the classic Dysfunctional Thoughts Record); checklists, questionnaires, and ratings; revisiting experiences in discussion with the therapist; and homework reviews. Reflection (including declarative knowledge) is encouraged by psychoeducation; formulation (see Chapter 3); relating the outcome of new experiences to previous ideas; drawing general conclusions and seeking alternative perspectives; reviewing progress; and summarizing learning, including the end-of-treatment relapse prevention package we call the patient's "therapy blueprint" (see Chapter 10). Planning is encouraged by identifying goals, objectives, and targets; agenda setting; design, preparation, and rehearsal of assignments; and action planning (including again the end-of-treatment "therapy blueprint"). Experience is encouraged by incorporating enactive methods into treatment and, par excellence, by making use of behavioral experiments.

For cognitive therapists, a beauty of the learning circle is that it maps directly on to the way behavioral experiments are designed, carried out, and evaluated in cognitive therapy. In addition, its potential breadth of reference means that it can be used not only to target anxiety, but to describe the process of learning through experience in a very wide range of conditions (see Bennett-Levy, Butler, et al., 2004). It provides a framework for working with cognitions at all levels of generality (from specific thoughts to broader, cross-situational assumptions and beliefs). This makes it potentially invaluable when working with multiple anxieties, anxiety comorbid with other Axis I disorders such as depression or eating disorders, and anxiety comorbid with long-standing problems such as interpersonal difficulties or low self-esteem. Thus, for patients, learning to use the circle as a means of structuring the learning process is a transferable skill with potential value for conducting behavioral experiments in a very wide range of problem areas.

CREATING SUCCESSFUL BEHAVIORAL EXPERIMENTS: THE PRACTICALITIES

The fundamental principles for creating effective behavioral experiments are the same across anxiety disorders, and indeed in relation to other associated problem areas reflected in comorbidity. The essential task, having identified a suitable target for investigation or testing (see Chapter 2), is to help the patient to follow through the sequence of processes encapsulated in the learning circle, that is, to use direct experience and self-reflection as a foundation for the acquisition of new knowledge and perspectives, an extended range of movement, and enduring change.

In this section we outline the steps involved in designing, carrying out, and evaluating effective behavioral experiments and follow with an extended clinical example (Alan). (Readers who would like further detail on the process should consult Rouf, Fennell, Westbrook, Cooper, & Bennett-Levy, 2004.) Our outline will take the form of helpful questions that therapists and patients can ask themselves at each stage, illustrating how guided discovery is central to the process. The answers to all these questions can only be found in consultation with the patient, and indeed the purpose of working together on designing and evaluating experiments is for patients to learn to do this for themselves. This is why it is important for therapist and patient to understand the principles involved in setting up effective behavioral experiments: The patient is not simply addressing the problem under immediate consideration but learning how to learn.

Planning Questions

- Is the purpose of the experiment clear? Is there a clear rationale?
- What are the target predictions? These may be straightforwardly expressed in words (e.g., "If I touch that frog, I will go screaming mad"), or they may take the form of an image (e.g., seeing and hearing what "going screaming mad" would be like), or a felt sense (e.g., a nameless dread). It is always worth inquiring about images, which are in effect sensory versions of verbal predictions, and remembering that they may be expressed through any of the senses, not just *visual* imagery (see Chapter 2). Patients may not report them spontaneously, especially if they are rapid snapshots rather than extended movies, but often recognize their presence if asked. The image can then be translated into words and rated for belief, or worked with as an image (see Chapter 5). Similarly, it is also worth explicitly inquiring about felt senses if they are not immediately reported, and investigating their meaning.
- What is the patient currently doing (or not doing) to ensure that the predictions do not come true (avoidance, safety-seeking behaviors)?
- How strongly does the patient believe the predictions (0–100%)? This rating will provide a baseline against which to measure change. Beliefs rarely go from 100% (present) to 0% (absent) in the course of a single experiment, and percentage ratings allow patient and therapist to acknowledge smaller changes.
- Is an alternative, more realistic, and/or positive prediction available? If so, what, and how strongly does the patient believe it? It is quite legitimate simply to test the existing point of view but can be helpful to specify an alternative (e.g., "If I touch this frog, I will be very anxious, but that's as far as it will go"). The experiment then becomes a test of competing hypotheses, and an opportunity to begin to establish and strengthen a new perspective. It is not always possible initially to find a viable alternative, especially if the patient believes the negative predictions 100%. However, even in this case, patients may be willing to accept alternatives formulated by their therapists, though their belief ratings are likely to be very low.
- How will the outcome of the experiment be evaluated? What outcome would sup-

port the negative prediction, and what outcome would contradict it? Equally, what outcome would support the new alternative, if there is one? It is important to inquire how the patient will know if the predictions have come true, especially in the case of interpersonal predictions where patients are often concerned not so much about what others will do as about how they will feel or what they will think. In this case, the therapist needs to inquire, for example: "How will you know if X thinks badly of you? How will they show that? What will they do that will tell you that that is what they are thinking?" An example can be found below in the description of Alan's sequence of experiments.

- What precisely will the patient do to test the prediction? If necessary, rehearse.
- Is the experiment manageable? That is, is it sufficiently challenging that new learning can occur, but not so challenging that the patient will be unable to carry it out?
- What difficulties might occur? How could these be prepared for?
- Has the experiment been set up as "no lose"? That is, is it clear that valuable information will be gained whether or not the outcome is as patient and therapist might hope? "Failed" experiments are often immensely valuable sources of information on what keeps the old system going, from which patient and therapist can learn.

Experience Questions

- Is the patient actually doing what she or he needs to do to test her or his predictions?
- Where is his or her attention focused? How far is he or she actually in touch with what is happening and looking out for signs that predictions have been confirmed or disconfirmed?
- Have safety-seeking behaviors been dropped? If the patient has the sense that she or he has had a lucky escape ("Phew! So far, so good"), then probably not.

Observation Questions (During and After the Experiment)

- What exactly is happening/happened? What do/did patient and therapist notice?
- What thoughts are/were present in the patient's mind? What is/was she or he feeling? What is/was happening in his or her body? What is she or he doing/did she or he do? How are/were others behaving?
- Were any old processing biases operating (e.g., screening out information that might disconfirm the prediction)? If so, what was their impact? Was the patient able to recognize and modify them at the time? And what happened then?

Reflection Questions

- What has the patient learned?
- How can his or her observations be understood? What do they mean?
- How does the outcome of the experiment relate to the original negative prediction? Does it confirm it, or contradict it? In the light of experience, how far does the patient now believe it (0–100%)?
- And how does the outcome relate to any more positive alternative that has been formulated? Does it confirm it, or contradict it? Again, rate for belief.
- If the negative prediction appears to have been confirmed, how might this be

accounted for? What does it mean? Does it follow that the patient was right and things will always be that way, or might it be that there was something about this specific situation which produced a negative outcome? For example, some people are bad tempered or rude when one talks to them. Many patients interpret this as a reflection of their own inadequacy, but actually it might be nothing to do with them—the grumpy person might be having a bad day, or be lacking in social skills, or there might be many other reasons for their behavior.

- How does the outcome of the experiment relate to the formulation as a whole? More specifically, what are its implications for the patient's broader dysfunctional assumptions, and beliefs about the self, others, and the world? Does it suggest that these perspectives are indeed correct, or that there might be room for doubt? When the patient keeps the outcome of the experiment in mind, how far does she or he believe the universal truth of these old ideas? Is it possible to formulate alternatives, however tentative, that seem better to fit what happened?
- How can what has been learned be carried over to different situations and across time (generalization)?
- What general principles about the process of change might be derived from this specific experience (e.g., "Things don't always work out as you hope, but that doesn't have to be the end of the world," "Doing experiments is scary, but it's worth it")?

Planning Questions (Preparing for the Next Experiment)

- What are the practical implications of new understanding derived from the last experiment?
- How can new learning be carried forward? What needs to be done next? Would it be best to consolidate learning by repeating the experiment, or to increase the level of risk by engaging in a more difficult situation? Or is further information needed? Or is it time to begin to explore a new area?
- And back to the beginning. What negative prediction is the patient aiming to test?

ALAN'S BEHAVIORAL EXPERIMENTS: A CLINICAL EXAMPLE

To see how conducting successful behavioral experiments plays out in practice, we next look at a sequence of experiments carried out by Alan early in therapy.

The starting point in the sequence was Alan's conviction that people were inherently dangerous and his anxiety that, if he approached them, they would immediately see him as monstrous and attack. The therapist suggested that a good way to begin testing these ideas might be a relatively unthreatening encounter with people he did not know well and would not have continued contact with—asking passers-by the way to a nearby shopping center. Alan was also afraid that what he feared would come true, but the therapist reassured him that she would be present to protect him and to provide encouragement and moral support, and reminded him of his wish not just to talk about the problem, but to do something about it. (She was personally convinced that the likelihood of physical attack or verbal abuse in response to such an innocuous question was virtually zero, given that the area where the experiment would be carried out was perfectly safe, it was the middle of the day, and most of the likely passers-by were local students and hospital workers.) Alan agreed to give it a try. His predictions were that, if he did so, 9 out of 10 people would despise him and tell him to shove off. One of the nine would be likely to attack him physically. These specific predictions (the entry point to the learning circle) were closely related to Alan's broader dysfunctional assumption ("If I approach people, they will attack me") and to his underlying beliefs about himself ("I am grotesque") and about others ("People are out to get me") (see Figure 6.1). Specific experiments would allow him to begin to chip away at these, even before they became targets in their own right.

Planning

Alan and his therapist worked out exactly what he would do when he encountered passers-by and how he would know if his predictions were true. He and the therapist rehearsed what he would say ("Excuse me, can you tell me the way to the shopping center please?"), and how to make eye contact (how else would he know how the person was reacting?) and if possible smile. It would be obvious if he was physically attacked, or if he was verbally abused, but the therapist was not clear how he would know that someone despised him. Alan said that they would have a particular ("sneering") look on their faces but could not describe in detail what he meant. So the therapist asked him to show her by doing it himself and then reflected it back to him so that they could be sure of exactly what they were looking for (lifted upper lip, frowning, corners of mouth pulled down, etc.). The therapist also pointed out that, given that she would be present, even if people did treat him rudely, they would be able to work out together what this might mean and if there was any way of making it less likely in the future.

Experience

When planning was complete, Alan and his therapist went out together. Their outing included a series of experiments, each building on the previous one, and each in miniature encapsulating the whole learning circle. Thus (as is often the case) experience was in fact interwoven with observation, reflection on the meaning of what had been observed, and planning the next step.

In the street outside the clinic they saw a young man approaching. When it came to the point, Alan said he simply couldn't do it. The therapist inquired if it was OK for her to do it for him, with him watching to see what reaction she got, and he agreed. So she asked the young man the way to the shopping center. The therapist observed that the man was perfectly civil, and Alan said that as far as he could tell nothing bad had happened. He pointed out that of course this might have been because the therapist had asked the way, rather than him. The therapist's response was to ask: "How could we find out if that is true?" and he admitted that this could only be discovered if he did the experiment himself. So he approached the next passer-by (a middle-aged woman) and asked her the way. Again, the therapist thought the response was perfectly civil, but when she asked what Alan had noticed, he said he did not know. He had been too apprehensive to look at the passer-by, and consequently had no real idea how she had responded. The therapist reassured him that this was quite understandable because he was doing something that felt extremely risky for the first time. He confirmed that his anxiety was at 110%. The therapist encouraged him ("You are doing a great job. I know this is really scary, and it's great that you have the courage to have a go"), and reminded him that unless he looked, he would not be able to discover anything useful or revise his predictions (reflection). They reviewed together what he would observe if his prediction was true (planning), and then he tried again (experience). This time Alan was able to observe the passer-by (a middle-aged man), and to notice that in fact there was no sign of sneering, abuse, or physical aggression (observation). Once again, the therapist reviewed the result, and congratulated him for his courage—and then it was on to planning and carrying out the next encounter.

Reflection

After Alan had successfully approached half a dozen people, the therapist called a temporary halt to the experiment and asked him what he made of the results so far (reflection). How well did what they had observed fit with his predictions? (It did not fit at all.) How consistent was it with his broader assumption about the dangers of approaching people? (It was not at all consistent.) And with his beliefs about himself, and them? (Again, not at all.) So what point of view might be more consistent with what had actually happened? The therapist asked him to keep the experiences he had just had center stage, and to see if he could find a new prediction that would better fit the facts as they had together observed them. After some um-ing and er-ing, Alan said tentatively: "Most people are OK and can be approached safely." The therapist went on to ask him what the people he met actually did that might fit this new idea. He said he didn't know what she meant, so she asked him specific clarifying questions: How did people stand? What about facial expression? What about tone of voice? And eye contact? And pace? In reflecting on these questions, Alan was able to recognize that people's stance had been open, relaxed, and facing toward him; that their expressions were friendly, smiling, or neutral at worst; that they had made eye contact; and that they did not rush past, but were willing to stop and take their time to make sure he understood their directions. This careful analysis meant that now, rather than simply testing Alan's old perspective, they could set the old and the new against one another in further experiments. Thus they would be able not just to undermine old ideas, but to strengthen still-fragile new ones.

Further In-Session Cycles

Alan and his therapist then reminded themselves what they might observe that would fit the original predictions (physical attack, verbal abuse, sneering expression) and the new perspective (open, smiling, etc.). This planning became the basis for a series of further encounters (repeatedly following through the steps of the circle), all of which produced results that supported the idea that most people are OK and can be approached safely. They then returned to the consulting room for an overall review of the afternoon.

Reflection

Alan said he now felt much less anxious about approaching people, and (if he held what had happened in mind) he could believe the new prediction 50%. He thought

What I did	"Asked the way to local shopping center—seven people. This meant making people notice me—including two women talking, man on cell phone."
What I predicted	"People would attack or verbally abuse me, or pay no attention to me."
Background ideas	"I am grotesque. People are out to get me, and will attack unless I avoid them."
Results	"All fine. Nothing bad came of it at all."
BUT	"Then I thought: 'I'm pushing my luck. Unless I stop now, something will happen.'"
	"My instinct was to stop—and that's what I would normally do. We realized this was a safety-seeking behavior, and if I stopped now I would be left with a feeling of 'near miss' and nothing would change—what I'd done would be wasted."
INSTEAD	"I pushed it. Even though I had to interrupt some people, and asked the way when a sign to the shopping center was right in front of us."
Results	"Talked to 21 people altogether. I thought in advance at least 4–5 of them would be angry and hostile—in fact, no one was. They were all friendly and helpful, or at worst neutral."
What I discovered	"People are not as scary as I thought. In fact, they are OK. Maybe that's not luck—it's how people really are. And I learned that it's OK to draw attention to myself."
What next?	"Carry on. Make eye contact, smile, and talk to lady in shop and man in garage. Watch like a hawk to see how they react. Write down what happens on sheet."

FIGURE 6.3. Summary of Alan's first sequence of behavioral experiments.

that before the sequence of experiments he would not have believed it at all. He still felt however that, once he was back in the real world, the new perspective would be hard to hold on to. So he and the therapist put their heads together and made a written summary that he would be able to consult as a reminder during the week (Figure 6.3).

Planning

As it was now the end of the session, the therapist asked Alan what he might be able to do before they met again that would allow him independently to build on what he had learned. At the thought of this, Alan felt nervous all over again. The therapist reassured him that he need not embark on the kind of intensive practice they had done together. For him to continue to build his confidence, it was important that he plan something that he felt he would be able to carry out successfully. If he overstretched himself, what would be likely to happen? Alan agreed that he would probably not be able to do as he had planned, and that this would be demoralizing. He decided that he would take the risk of making eye contact, smiling, and speaking briefly to the woman behind the counter at his local grocery store, and to the man at the fuel station on his way home from work. He felt it would be possible to do this once for each person during the week. He would do his best to watch their reactions, and decide whether they fit the old perspective or the new. The therapist talked him through the behavioral experiments record sheet (Figure 6.4), and they agreed that he would record his experiments on the sheet.

Date	Problem Situation What is the issue I am tackling?	Prediction(s) What exactly do I think will happen unless I take precautions? What is the worst that might happen? How would I know if it did?	Experiment What will I do to test the prediction? (e.g., facing a situation I would normally avoid, dropping precautions, behaving in a new way)	Outcome What actually happened? Was my prediction correct?	What I learned

FIGURE 6.4. Record sheet for behavior experiments.

MAXIMIZING THE IMPACT OF BEHAVIORAL EXPERIMENTS

Working to a Realistic Time Scale

Alan's difficulties were long term and substantial, and a sequence of small-scale experiments of this kind would not on its own revolutionize his thinking or radically change his approach to life. However, the process of planning, experience, observation, reflection, and thinking ahead to the next step allowed the introduction of doubt: It became possible to begin to entertain the idea that his fears (though entirely understandable, given his experiences) were in fact inaccurate, and that there might be more helpful and realistic possibilities to be investigated. What Alan discovered in these first experiments became the foundation for a gradual, extended process of exploration in situations he perceived as increasingly threatening.

Being able to manage everyday encounters with ease—and even to appreciate and enjoy such little moments of human warmth—is a radical step for someone as frightened as Alan. However, it is only the first step to something more difficult: taking the risk of allowing people closer, of opening up with people with whom he would normally be highly defensive and avoidant, especially women. Alan was able to identify a small number of social situations in which he felt able to relax (all with people that he knew very well), and this provided a tiny glimpse of how things might possibly develop with others. However, this was necessarily a long-term project, and anticipating and working through setbacks would be an important part of it.

Using the Results of Behavioral Experiments to Develop the Formulation

Experiments not only create new opportunities for patients, but also contribute to their understanding of how their own personal belief systems work (metacognitive awareness; Chapter 4). They provide access to material that may not be accessible in the safety of the consulting room, for instance, revealing detail about the sequencing of elements in maintaining cycles that is difficult to map out accurately without direct observation. This is because exposure to real situations can trigger emotions and appraisals that are hard to get hold of, or easy to rationalize away, when patients are at some distance from what they fear.

During the series of experiments described above, for example, the therapist picked up on an issue she had observed when Alan approached his first passer-by, and at the beginning of every therapy session: Alan's failure to look at the person he was talking to. Even though they had now met on a number of occasions, and Alan seemed to have some confidence in the work they were doing together, each time the therapist went to meet him in the waiting room, he avoided eye contact and gave no nonverbal signs of greeting or recognition (smiling, etc.). Instead, he tended to speak gruffly and scowl. The therapist was aware that her own response was to feel rather rejected and want to pull away, and she suspected that this might also be the reaction of other people Alan encountered. So in the following session she asked Alan to consider how his fears about others might affect how he behaved with them, what messages he might unintentionally convey, and how this might affect encounters. Together, on the whiteboard, they elaborated the initial formulation, detailing the toxic maintaining cycle ("old system") which is captured in the inner circle of Figure 6.5. What typically came to Alan's mind when he met someone new? And how did he then feel? And what did he do to stop the predictions from coming true? And what kind of message might that behavior unwittingly give to the other person? What might *they* then do? And what was the impact of that on what he thought in the first place?

Then, step by step, they considered how the new perspective might affect his behavior with others and, in turn, their responses to him. This is mapped out in the outer circle of Figure 6.5. Supposing he was able to believe the new idea that most people are OK and can be approached safely, what would then come to mind when he met one? And how would he then feel? And so on. The "old system" (inner circle) was written in black, and the "new system" (outer circle) was written in green, so that the differences stood out clearly. Because it was on the whiteboard, they could keep changing it until Alan felt it fit, and ensure that it was in his words. He and the therapist then made copies for themselves on paper, with each circle in a different colored ink, so that they could use it to guide future experiments.

It should be noted that the information included in this elaboration is not all entirely new—Figure 6.1, derived at the beginning of treatment, shows that some elements had already been identified through earlier discussions and observations. However, the elaboration allowed cognitive, affective, and behavioral elements and their interpersonal consequences to be clearly, logically, and economically related to one

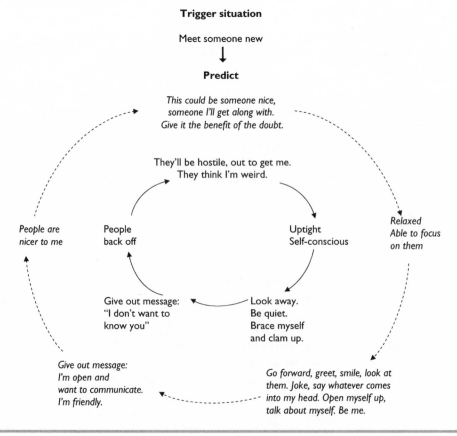

FIGURE 6.5. Old system, new system (Alan).

another, and used as a basis for new alternatives that Alan would have found utterly alien at the beginning of treatment.

Using the Therapeutic Relationship

In cognitive therapy, the therapeutic relationship is crucially important. Establishing and maintaining rapport creates a framework within which therapist and patient can fruitfully work together, and therapy cannot proceed productively without some degree of trust on both sides. This is perhaps particularly essential in relation to behavioral experiments, which necessarily require patients to take what they feel to be substantial risks. However, as the eye-contact example illustrates, glitches and ruptures in the therapeutic relationship can provide vital "live" information (validated in Alan's case by observations during experiments) that therapist and patient can explore together and use as a basis for change, not only in what happens between them, but also elsewhere (Leahy, 2001; Safran & Muran, 2000; Safran & Segal, 1990). In addition, it is interesting to speculate on how therapists' willingness to do things that patients perceive as frightening, on their behalf (as happened when the therapist approached the first passer-by), may enhance the therapeutic relationship. In fact, provided a good relationship has been established, in-session behavioral experiments are often energizing and even fun.

Providing an Objective Eye

At least during early sessions, patients may be too anxious and self-preoccupied while doing experiments to be able to see clearly what is going on (as was Alan when he first approached a passer-by himself). On other occasions, even when they are not as anxiously preoccupied, well-practiced processing biases may come into play and make it difficult for them to view the situation as might a dispassionate observer. Conducting experiments during the therapy session means that the therapist is at hand to help the patient to reach a more objective perspective. She or he can provide prompts to detached observation (e.g., "Look at his face—what do you notice? What's the expression?") and reflection (e.g., "What do you make of that? Is that your old fears speaking?"). This helps the patient to tune into what is actually happening, instead of biasing incoming information in line with preexisting ideas, and to be able to relate what is observed to initial predictions, broader assumptions and beliefs, and emerging new perspectives, so that useful conclusions may be drawn and the ground prepared for the next stage. With experience, patients learn to ask themselves questions of this kind.

Spotting Residual Safety-Seeking Behaviors

Equally, therapists can be alert for doubts and reservations about the validity of findings, and the subtle safety-seeking behaviors that often underlie them. These habitual precautions may be so well ingrained that patients are only minimally (if at all) aware of them.

An example occurred during the series of experiments described above. After seven encounters, Alan announced that he thought it had been enormously useful to do these experiments, and he had learned a huge amount, so there was little point in continuing, and could they go back to the consulting room now. The therapist would have loved to believe that this was true—a miracle cure! However, she was also suspicious, so she asked him what was going through his mind. Alan replied: "I don't want to push my luck." "How do you mean, exactly?" asked the therapist. It turned out that he believed that it was pure chance that nothing bad had happened up to that point, but if he continued then hostile reactions were sure to follow. Had he been on his own, he would have gone home at that point. The therapist said that she was delighted he had said what he did—now they could see just how powerful and sneaky the old system was. She asked: "How can we test that out?" and Alan ruefully agreed that there was only one way: more experiments. With her continuing praise and encouragement, he proceeded to approach a further 14 people, including what Alan saw as instances where hostility was particularly likely (where, e.g., he had to interrupt because people were talking to one another, or speaking on their cell phones). Still nothing happened.

Alan then said that perhaps this was because instructions for reaching the shopping center (which was just around the corner) were very short and straightforward. If something more complex and time-consuming was required, then surely his prediction would come true. Again, the therapist's response was "How can we test that out?" In a follow-up series of experiments, during the next therapy session, they went to a busy intersection and asked passers-by the way to a hospital that was at some distance and required complex directions. The test was made more rigorous by the fact that it was raining. Nonetheless, people responded helpfully and were willing to take the time to answer Alan's question. In fact, one passer-by said that he was going there himself and suggested that they go together. It took some ingenuity on the therapist's part to extricate them from this situation.

Generalizing from Specific Experiments

Alan's experiments affected his cognitions at different levels of generality. He tested highly specific predictions ("If I ask *this particular person* the way, *he* will attack me"), and also to begin to chip away at his broader assumption ("If I approach *anyone*, *that person* will attack me"), and his central beliefs that he was grotesque and others' aggressive. Multilevel change of this kind (illustrated diagrammatically with an example from another patient in Figure 6.6) is facilitated by questions like, "How does what we have observed here relate to your general sense that, if approached, people are going to attack you?" and "How do the reactions you have received this morning relate to your idea about yourself as grotesque? Have people responded as if that was true?" Thus the work of weakening old assumptions and beliefs can begin even while the prime target is situation-specific cognitive, affective, and behavioral change.

Speeding up Learning

Patients may feel able, with the support of the therapist, to go further than they would dare to go on their own. This potentially increases the speed of learning. For example, Alan wanted to do a course in bookkeeping at his local community college but was nervous about asking for details of what was available. During a later therapy session, he and his therapist visited the college and went to the registration office. After asking a

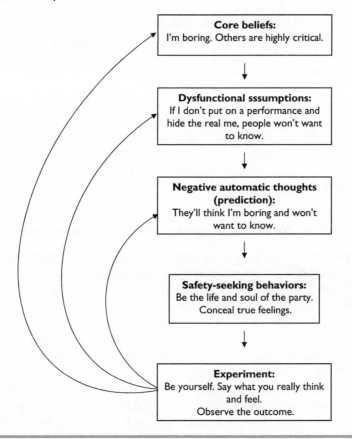

FIGURE 6.6. Behavioral experiments and multilevel change.

couple of questions, Alan turned to leave. The therapist suspected that this was pretty much what he would normally have done, and that it might be useful to push things further. As it was not possible with office staff close by to discuss this with Alan, she decided unilaterally to say that she was interested in the same course and asked a long series of questions (sometimes repeating herself), which took some time to answer. The receptionist remained polite and friendly. Afterwards, Alan admitted that he had wanted to know more but had not dared to ask. He had had no idea that it was possible to draw things out at such length without adverse consequences.

Deconstructing the Old, or Constructing the New?

For some patients, especially those with recurrent problems and major interpersonal difficulties, it has been suggested that deconstructing the old system may be less productive than creating a new system (a new self) and operating from that (Mooney & Padesky, 2000). Chadwick, Birchwood, and Trower (1996) proposed that "beliefs rarely change as a result of intellectual challenging, but only through engaging emotions and behaving in new ways that produce evidence that confirms new beliefs" (p. 37).

This was true for Alan. Homing in on his old beliefs and assumptions to weaken them produced a dramatic shift in mood because it put him in contact with painful memories, his sense of a life wasted, and deep hopelessness. He became seriously depressed and even suicidal over the course of a week. This deeply concerned the therapist, who suggested that perhaps it would be more helpful to take the tentative new perspective as a template (the outer circle of Figure 6.4), work from that, and observe the outcome. Alan agreed with relief, his sense of cautious optimism returned, and his mood improved. For many people, deconstructing the old is an extremely valuable aspect of therapy and a useful prelude to constructing and strengthening the new. Therapists should be aware, however, that at times this work can be unproductive or actively unhelpful (perhaps especially with people whose early experiences have profoundly undermined their sense of their own identity), and be prepared to move flexibly to focusing primarily on establishing and strengthening new alternatives.

Interweaving Behavioral Experiments with Other Interventions

Behavioral experiments are a crucial part of working with anxiety, but they are not the full story. Continuing experiments, in session and for homework, were interwoven for Alan with other interventions, including finding a potential alternative to his sense of himself ("I am a normal human being, but things that have happened in my life have made me see myself as grotesque"); encouraging him to start noticing and giving weight to aspects of his daily life that endorsed the idea that he was a normal human being ("positive data logging"; Padesky, 1994); obtaining feedback from other people on how he actually came over to them, especially when relatively relaxed and externally focused (nervous and shy, but a nice man about whom they would like to know more); helping him to take better care of himself with regular exercise, time to relax, and a healthier diet. Thus experiments are only part of a much more varied program of interventions.

THERAPIST-GUIDED IN-SESSION EXPERIMENTS

Alan admitted after his first venture into behavioral experiments that, if he had had to do this on his own, he would undoubtedly have been too terrified and "chickened out." This observation captures a key benefit of conducting experiments in session, in the presence of the therapist.

Therapist-guided behavioral interventions, carried out within session, are an integral part of behavior therapy (e.g., going out and about with agoraphobics, or treating OCD in the home so as to ensure effective exposure and response prevention). Many cognitive therapists, in contrast, see patients only in their consulting rooms and rarely venture out into the real world. Behavioral experiments are still interwoven with cognitive interventions, but the usual pattern (if therapists attending workshops on the topic are to be believed) is that they are mostly (or indeed entirely) carried out independently by patients, as between-session homework assignments. It is not difficult to see why this might be the case: In-session experiments take time and may require resources that are difficult to access (video cameras, audiences, wildlife, elevators, etc.). Therapists may be concerned about the insurance implications, or feel that they cannot afford the longer sessions behavioral experiments often require, especially when they involve leaving the consulting room.

We would strongly argue that a single 1½- or 2-hour session with a well-targeted experiment, or series of experiments, may save a number of hours of discussion and failed intervening homework assignments. "Homework compliance" is a perennial clinical stumbling block in cognitive therapy. Consider your own experience as a therapist: Can you say, with your hand on your heart, that you have *never* had the experience of agreeing an assignment with a patient, only to have the patient return the following week without having carried it out at all, having carried it out in a state of anxiety so acute that they have been unable clearly to observe what happened or consider what it meant, or with it having "gone wrong" with resultant distress and demoralization? The key question may be, not "Can I afford to put in the extra time and organization needed?" but rather "Can I afford *not* to?"

CONCLUSION

We said that the most effective method of learning is direct experience—behavioral experiments, built on a foundation of careful assessment and formulation work, and closely linked with cognitions central to problem development and maintenance. Behavioral experiments stimulate curiosity (rather than a need to control), provide opportunities to welcome and take advantage of the unexpected (rather than fearing it), open new avenues for learning by encouraging us to approach what we might prefer to avoid, and teach us to respond to events with flexibility (rather than rigidity and constriction). Now is your chance to find this out for yourself. As Judith Beck (1995) observed in relation to recording negative thoughts (p. 127), clinicians would do well to master cognitive therapy methods themselves, using their own concerns, before attempting to teach them to patients. We invite you to use this opportunity to explore the method for yourself, using a genuine anxiety of your own to discover the potential power and pitfalls of behavioral experiments designed according to the Learning Circle before returning to using them with patients.

It is fine to do this work on your own. However, it may enrich your learning to do it with a colleague or friend, someone you trust and who is willing to experiment too. You can then act as each other's "therapist" and "patient" and help each other to make the most of experiments, just as you would in treatment with a real patient. You will find in Figures 6.7 and 6.8 worksheets for planning and evaluating your own behavioral experiments. We suggest that you record what you do on these sheets (which also offer an alternative format for patients to record their own experiments). You can also use the questions on pages 114–116 above to structure your investigation.

We hope that you will find this intriguing, challenging, and an opportunity for genuine personal learning and growth, as well as a chance to use self-practice and self-reflection to enhance your therapeutic skills (Bennett-Levy, 2006) and, not least, to appreciate the extraordinary courage our patients show when they allow us to persuade them to embark on behavioral experiments. As one highly experienced clinician observed in a workshop after carrying out a personally relevant behavioral experiment: "I'm glad I tried it out with a real issue—something that really does bother me. I never realized how terrifying it is to put yourself on the line like that. I have been telling patients to go out and do behavioral experiments for years without a second thought. I shall take more care in future. I had no idea how much courage it takes."

I. Identify your target for change

Select an issue you would genuinely like to work on, that is, something that you would normally avoid because of anxiety, or do only with precautions (safety-seeking behaviors) in place. This could be something as simple as picking up a spider, or as complicated as being newly assertive with someone who intimidates you. Don't forget things that might benefit your patients, but which you would have difficulty with (e.g., pretending to faint or vomit in public).

2. Identify your predictions

Identify the negative predictions that lead you to avoid, or to use precautions (thoughts, images, "felt sense"). What if you did not? What is the worst that might happen? Rate your belief in the predictions (0–100%).

Do you have an alternative, more positive prediction as well? If so, rate belief in that too.

Can you identify broader issues that your specific predictions might reflect (assumptions, beliefs)?

3. Identify an experiment

Identify a specific behavioral experiment that will allow you to test your predictions. Decide when and where you will carry it out.

What exactly will you do that you normally would not (avoidance), or not do that you normally would (safety-seeking behaviors)? What safety-seeking behaviors will you drop? What will you do instead?

How will you assess the outcome of the experiment? What will you look out for? What might you observe that would confirm your negative predictions? And what would contradict them? If you have a positive alternative, what would confirm that or contradict it?

FIGURE 6.7. Design your own experiment: Planning.

1. Observation

What exactly happened? What did you do (or not do)? What did you notice (thoughts, feelings, body sensations, environment, other people)? Were there any difficulties? What did you do about them?

2. Reflection

What have you learned? How can you make sense of what you observed? What does it mean?

How do your observations relate to your negative predictions? Do they confirm or contradict them? If the latter, what perspective might make more sense? And how do your observations relate to any more positive predictions you had?

What have you discovered about behavioral experiments (the principles)?

3. Planning

Personal implications of the experiment
What you have learned about yourself? How could you build on that, and carry it forward? What next?

Professional implications of the experiment
How can you use what you have learned with patients? How will you integrate what you have discovered in your clinical practice? What is the first step? When will you use your new learning, and with whom?

FIGURE 6.8. Design your own experiment: Observation, reflection, and planning.

PART IV

OVERCOMING THREE MAJOR OBSTACLES TO PROGRESS

"I don't really know what I feel."
"Everyone else can handle this. What's wrong with me that I can't?"
"But something dreadful could happen at any time."

In this part of the book we consider three separate difficulties that can interfere with progress even when standard treatment for anxiety is skillfully applied. These obstacles usually reflect long-standing cognitive-affective patterns with strong links to behavior, and their effects may be apparent not only in the later stages, but also throughout treatment. They may make it hard for patients to engage with treatment, slow down the course of change, and/or increase the likelihood of relapse.

In Chapter 7, "Avoidance of Affect," we focus on the fear of having, expressing, or being on the receiving end of strong feelings. These fears can apply to all feelings (even to positive ones), and usually people have their own good reasons for such fears. In this chapter we define the problem, discuss how to recognize and make sense of it, and then provide a range of practical methods for overcoming it.

Chapter 8 recognizes that anxiety often coexists with *low self-esteem*. This can be understood either as a contributory cause of the anxiety or as one of its consequences, and it often lies at the heart of comorbidity with depression, with other Axis I conditions, and with personality disorder. A cognitive model of low self-esteem provides a coherent way of understanding the problem, and a basis for treating it effectively and efficiently.

Finally in Chapter 9, "Dealing with Uncertainty," we bring together the main themes running through this book by focusing on ways of developing attitudes for the future that allow us all to consider facing the unknown more with equanimity, interest, or curiosity than with anxiety.

Each of the chapters in this part of the book is filled with practical methods for resolving the problems arising from these difficulties, and although specific research is not currently available, our understanding is that when such obstacles are removed patients are then able to take advantage of the standard methods for treating anxiety that are demonstrably so effective. A general strategy for approaching obstacles to treatment is also demonstrated in these chapters. This involves careful observation to define the difficulty, making sense of it in terms of current theory and case formulation work, and then using this understanding as a basis for considering treatment options and possible pitfalls.

SEVEN

Avoidance of Affect

Avoidance of affect is one of the cognitive-affective patterns that, especially when it is long-standing, interferes with progress, and which in practice is at first hard to recognize. Attempts to avoid internal experiences, such as thoughts, feelings, or sensations, have been shown to occur across anxiety disorders. They have also been shown to play a part in the maintenance of disorders (Harvey et al., 2004; Hayes, Wilson, Strosahl, Gifford, & Follette, 1996). Thus if they continue so will the problems that give rise to the disorders. In this chapter we focus on recognizing, understanding, and finding ways of overcoming attempts to avoid one of these internal experiences: feelings (or affect).

Despite some initial reticence or embarrassment, most people who seek treatment for anxiety are able to describe their difficulties and to talk about their problems, especially when an accepting therapist facilitates the process of disclosure. However, there is a subset of people who find this extremely difficult: those who avoid affect. People who avoid feelings and emotions try to protect themselves from affective experiences and often reduce the perceived risk by using safety-seeking behaviors. They usually avoid experiencing them and expressing them, and they may avoid provoking the experience and the expression of feelings in others as well. In extreme cases feelings in all their manifestations have become a major source of threat, and the possibility of experiencing them, showing them, talking about them, or eliciting them in others induces the felt sense of vulnerability that is the hallmark of anxiety. People may then adopt a self-protective mode of living that affects them in numerous ways, some of which are described below (see also Butler & Surawy, 2004).

> Douglas was a car mechanic in a large garage. The others working there gossiped, joked, and laughed as they worked. Douglas felt like a complete outsider. He tried to join in by being funny, but his jokes fell flat, and then he was teased. No one asked him to join them at break times, or for a drink after work. He tried not to react to being left out, and to be "deadpan" so that his feelings did not show. He pretended that he did not care. A similar thing happened when he found a girlfriend. He pretended that he had a busy social life and ended up alone on occasions when he could have been with her. Douglas had been his father's favorite child. He had two older stepbrothers (also his father's children) who he admired

greatly. They were big and strong when he was small; they had lively friends with whom they played football; later on they had girlfriends and went out a lot. But they resented their father's treatment of Douglas and ostracized him. Douglas believed that he was weird, different, and unacceptable, and his main strategy when with other people was to try to be whatever he thought they wanted him to be—and to hide his feelings away.

Patients' reports suggest that when avoiding, or seeking safety from emotional arousal, their attention is diverted toward other aspects of experience such as activities, achievements, verbal behavior, or physical sensations. A significant subgroup pay attention to physiological rather than psychological aspects of emotion, and their cognitions focus correspondingly on the meaning of bodily changes (e.g., "there's something wrong"), sensations and discomfort, and on the meaning to them of these changes (e.g., "I could be ill").

> Julie was the manager of a warehouse. Her work started early, and she worked late most nights as well. She found it easier to get things done when there were few other people around, and she organized her life around routines that meant she "never had to stop and think," to plan ahead, or to worry about making big decisions. She took her responsibilities seriously and had been unable to make up her mind about whether to join her new partner for a holiday. In the end he went without her and then broke off the relationship. Julie tried not to think about it and worked even harder. Three months later she visited her doctor saying that she had been unable to get rid of the aftereffects of a bad cold and still had persistent headaches. She was worried about them and requested a brain scan. She found it upsetting to hear that there could be a psychological component to her symptoms and could not at first consider this as a real possibility.

For such people the content of underlying beliefs (e.g., "It's wrong to let your feelings show") is likely to be closely linked to their fear of affect so that activating, or threatening to activate, these beliefs will be associated with intense distress. Then people go out of their way to avoid doing or saying anything that feels even slightly emotional, and a hint of anger, or of friendliness, may be sufficient to trigger a massive retreat. Avoidance may be so rapid and effective that it is hard for patients subsequently to recount their experiences to others, for example, during therapy.

Common consequences of avoidance of affect include difficulties in forming and keeping relationships, being unable to act so as to meet personal goals, low self-esteem (which is discussed in the next chapter), and increases in physical, as opposed to psychological, symptoms. It can be particularly difficult to form intimate relationships. Because the problem interferes with the ability to relate to others and to do things with them, it can prevent people achieving many kinds of personal goals.

> Martin was a talker. He could easily fill each session with interesting and lively but entirely superficial discussion. He described his mother as a storyteller who could entertain people for hours. But he never touched on his own feelings, and he lived an isolated and lonely existence. He was unable to accept an offer of promotion for fear of having to develop new ways of relating to people. He longed for an intimate relationship but could only communicate with people as his "real self" when

using the Internet. One of his first goals was to reduce his compulsive and time-consuming use of the computer.

The tendency to avoid feelings sometimes develops following painful experiences that have not been fully processed, and the possibility of thinking about these can be filled with dread. Starting to do so provokes distressing intrusions (memories, thoughts, images, and nightmares as described in Chapter 5), which seem to confirm that it is preferable to continue living in self-protective mode, and advisable to keep a tight hold on emotions: to keep the experience and the expression of them at bay. Understandably these reactions can interfere with the straightforward application of standard methods of treatment, including those described in detail in Chapter 5.

Typical surface-level cognitions reflect an element of uncertainty and are often rather vague: "If this goes on, I'll lose it." "This feels horrible, I need to get away." The possibility of developing close relationships with others, within therapy as well as outside it, feels uncomfortable and may trigger anxiety-provoking predictions: "I'll be shown up" and "I won't be able to handle this." Some people find these hard to put into words, or feel ashamed of doing so, and then their attempts may sound less like the report of a thought than a description of a "felt sense" that occurs when they are exposed to something strange and alarming.

TRANSDIAGNOSTIC FEATURES OF AVOIDANCE OF AFFECT

Avoidance of affect occurs in many disorders but is especially common in avoidant personality disorder, social anxiety, and health anxiety, and in each case it has somewhat different manifestations. In avoidant personality disorder it appears to be part of the general, pervasive pattern of avoidance described in the DSM (for a detailed account of this, see Padesky & Beck, 2003); in social anxiety it may be more closely associated with the fear of being judged (and found wanting) by other people—by the fear of negative evaluation, and in health anxiety emotions are sometimes manifested more readily in physical than in psychological ways. In addition, it is often described by people who have suffered from abuse, violence, or emotional neglect, and by some with binge-eating disorder (who may have had similar experiences). Avoiding schema activation, which can occur in any of the personality disorders, may be another manifestation of avoidance of affect. Young and colleagues (2003), when describing their concept of schema modes, said that "the Detached Protector mode is characterized by the absence of emotion, combined with high levels of avoidance" (p. 41). The emotional numbing that commonly follows a traumatic incident, and the reluctance to think or talk about past traumatic or painful experiences, may be similar phenomena.

People who are especially anxious about upsetting significant others, for example, people with agoraphobia (Chambless & Goldstein, 1982; Hackmann, 1998a) may go out of their way to avoid provoking negative feelings in them. This, however, reflects just one aspect of avoidance of affect, as it may go hand in hand with needing to please and to elicit positive feelings from others, and may not be so closely associated with efforts to avoid the (personal) experience of affect.

Despite the different contexts in which avoidance of affect occurs, and the supposedly different reasons for it, there are ways of understanding it and of helping people to overcome it that have more general application, and these are the focus of this chapter.

Reduced affect also occurs in psychopathy and narcissism, but in these cases it is conceptualized in terms of poor empathy rather than avoidance and will therefore not be discussed further here. We explain and illustrate what we mean by avoidance of affect first and then go on to consider ways of making sense of it and ways of helping people to become less fearful of their own feelings and those of others.

THE MEANING OF AFFECT

Chapter 2, which describes how to explore cognitions in depth, started with a reminder of the theory underpinning cognitive therapy, which "postulates that emotional disturbance is triggered by appraisals accessible via the contents of consciousness, which include thoughts and images. Affect is considered to be an important 'marker' that indicates the presence of relevant appraisals" (p. 30). If this account is correct, then avoiding affect will make it harder for patients to reflect on cognitive as well as affective activity, and it will be difficult for them to identify all levels of cognition: thoughts, assumptions, and beliefs. Therapists may also find it difficult to develop specific hypotheses to make sense of their patients' problems. So formulation work may be less straightforward than usual, and the process of therapy may feel stilted, impoverished, or awkward. Although people probably avoid affect for their own good reasons, some of which will be discussed below (pp. 137–138), the underlying theme is that they do so because they find emotions disturbing. So it is important briefly to consider why avoiding, or suppressing, feelings would matter: to think about the meaning, and the value to us all of having feelings.

In his book *The Evolution of Consciousness*, Ornstein (1991) argued strongly for the evolutionary value of emotions:

> The pivot of the internal self is emotion. This dominant "self-ish" brain lies in frontal lobe and limbic system linkages that appraise threats in the environment and organise quick actions. Human beings can override this usual mode of operation: actions can be reconsidered, we can learn and grow from experiences, conscious control can modify ineffective tendencies. But most often and most reliably, especially in eras long gone, feeling our way through worked best. (p. 153)

Not only do we need our feelings, but we can (or at least could in eras long gone) rely on them in ways that conferred advantage. We save ourselves by running away when in danger but might not do so if we were not scared. We are more likely to prolong the species if we respond to our feelings of affection by seeking to be close to someone we love. As Gilbert (2005a) argued, our feelings of compassion for others contribute to the social glue that binds members of a society together. Arguably, there is a sense in which emotion is primary.

In the second place, emotions provide us with information. Psychologists' models of multilevel information-processing systems (e.g., Barnard & Teasdale, 1991; Brewin et al., 1996; Dalgleish & Power, 1999) suggested ways in which emotion and cognition interact and contribute to the various processes involved, including attention, interpretation, storage, and retrieval. Despite differences between these theories, there appears to be a consensus that emotion and cognition must be considered to construct a plausible account of information-processing systems. This would help to explain why (as described by Goleman, 1996, in an account of work by Damasio) people who are unable to access emotional information following specific damage to links between the limbic system and prefrontal lobes find it hard to make decisions. One might assume that it would be easier to make decisions if one could weigh the pros and cons dispassionately and analytically, but without access to affect it is not even easy to decide which are the pros and which the cons. Emotion provides the color that helps us to differentiate one set of conditions from another, so to speak, and without it it is much harder to make decisions (to plan ahead and to organize ourselves so as to meet our needs), and to interact well with others. Hence, contemporary theories of emotion emphasize its adaptive value (Gross, 1998; Mayer, Salovey, Caruso, & Sitarenios, 2003).

A third point is that all of us learn to modulate our expressions of emotion according to what is socially appropriate and acceptable within our individual contexts and cultures. Emotions may be essential and informative, but displaying them inappropriately, by bursting into tears or exploding with anger at work or in a restaurant, for instance, has unpleasant social repercussions such as shame or embarrassment and risks provoking an unsympathetic response from others.

However, continuing to avoid will maintain current difficulties, whereas exposure will reduce them.

> Exposure is the key to most change ... exposure in its many forms is central to both intrapersonal and interpersonal change. In psychodynamic thinking, anxiety and avoidance are central to repression, the treatment of which involves "uncovering" (exposing patients to) feared images, emotions, and/or thoughts often in a stepwise fashion ... Exposure seems to mean "controlled exposure to reality" so that new information helps to correct old distorted schemas. (Beitman, 1992, pp. 205–206)

There is no alternative but to face the fears; and, as illustrated in Chapter 6, an effective way to do this is to use well-constructed behavioral experiments. These provide a cognitive framework for the exposure that assists in ensuring the relevance of new information and provide a method for considering this new information alongside old ways of seeing things: "so that new information helps to correct old distorted schema" and can speed up the process of recovery. Recent work on social phobia (Clark et al., 2006) and on agoraphobia (Salkovskis et al., 2007) provides evidence that a good outcome is achieved with less exposure when the exposure is provided in a cognitive context. But first it is important to consider how to recognize avoidance of affect, as this is not always easy.

RECOGNIZING AVOIDANCE OF AFFECT

To recognize avoidance of affect it is important to pay close attention to the moment-to-moment process of therapy, to tune in to how far it is possible to develop a sense of connectedness, and to consider the appropriateness of any emotions expressed to the topics being discussed. The usual advice to cognitive therapists is to look for "hot" cognitions, paying close attention to signs of emotional arousal. The assumption is that the "hotter" the emotion the more likely that significant core beliefs or schema are activated, making it easier to develop useful formulations and to decide where to focus the work of searching for alternative perspectives. When avoidance of affect is habitual and pervasive the opposite pattern can occur, so that the possibility of activating (painful) beliefs or schema is accompanied by increasing loss of affect. Then the trail becomes colder, not hotter, the closer you get to heart of the matter. There are numerous different signs of avoidance of affect, and many of these can also be attributed to other factors. Some of the more common signs are listed below.

- Gaze changes, reduced eye contact.
- Fidgeting and changing body position.
- Changing the topic; distracting attention to something else.
- Intellectualizing; engaging others in interesting discussions.
- Ruminating; worrying.
- Telling jokes or diverting anecdotes.
- Appearing not to understand.
- Withdrawing or "shutting down."
- Skillful ways of keeping other people talking.
- Indecisiveness.
- Going blank, disengaging, forgetting, dissociating.
- Binge eating, drinking, drug taking, or deliberate self-harm.

Although it is sometimes clear, particularly from the tone of therapy, that someone finds emotional arousal disturbing, many sources of ambiguity remain and can make the task of recognizing the problem difficult. For example, the borderlines between privacy, secrecy, and avoidance are hard to define, and there are cultural differences in the kinds of feelings that it is acceptable to talk about or to show. Answers to straightforward questions about the kinds of feelings that are generally acceptable in a person's current or childhood context, or in a particular situation, are often informative in that they help the therapist to understand which kinds of feelings (shame, anger, disappointment, affection, for instance) are likely to elicit and to maintain anxiety and avoidance. Validating the wishes of someone (especially someone who has not been treated well previously) to choose what to share and what not to share, can help, but not always. It can be useful to discuss the pros and cons of expressing feelings, and to encourage people to experiment with disclosing more feelings within and outside therapy. In addition, there is also the problem of denial. For some people this appears to be a functional strategy when faced with distressing information (evidence of the malignant behavior of a parent, or a diagnosis of terminal illness, for instance). We should not assume that "being in denial" is always harmful, but be ready to think about its advantages and disadvantages in particular cases or situations.

MAKING SENSE OF AVOIDANCE OF AFFECT: THEORIES, CAUSES, AND CONSEQUENCES

In practice the most useful starting point for making sense of avoidance of affect in an individual case is to ascertain the meaning to the person of having, expressing, or provoking feelings. Often this is not easy to do. For people who minimize or deny feelings, admitting that feelings are overwhelming, for instance, may itself be an overwhelming experience. For them the threshold for feeling overwhelmed is also likely to be low (they may generally adopt a repressive coping style; Brewin, 1997). One way out of this difficulty is to take advantage (temporarily) of the skill of the patient who avoids affect in talking about, rather than having feelings, and to keep the conversational tone light—or humorous. The Tin Man in *The Wizard of Oz* may be a useful example to draw upon. Feelings may be seen, for example, as:

- Overwhelming, unmanageable, uncontrollable.
- Unacceptable, shameful, humiliating.
- Childish, weak, immature.
- Inappropriate.
- Dangerous.

These meanings may apply to some feelings, or to all feelings, positive or negative. They may apply to one's own feelings and/or to those of others. They often involve all or nothing patterns of thinking about feelings.

Three additional sources of information that contribute to the understanding of avoidance of affect are described next: theoretical ideas, hypotheses about causes, and information about the consequences of avoidance of affect.

Theoretical Considerations

Anxiety supposedly arises when perceived threats outweigh perceived resources (internal and external) for dealing with them. When affect is generally avoided people are thus likely to become hypervigilant for the sensations associated with emotional arousal or for indicators of emotional arousal in others, and to overestimate the degree of risk or threat involved. They may also underestimate their personal resources for dealing with emotional experiences or displays, and for keeping their feelings hidden or within the supposed limits of (personal or cultural) acceptability.

Butler and Surawy (2004) suggested that three kinds of cognitive biases are likely to be associated with avoidance of affect. First, attentional biases determine what is noticed: inner tension, changes in heart rate, the body posture or facial expressions of others. Second, interpretations are consistent with underlying attitudes: "This feels risky" and "Something unpleasant is going to happen next." Third, selective and state-dependent memory confirm and endorse the biases: remembering being ignored when upset, or being bullied for being too serious; memories of receiving a cold and rejecting response when distressed; or the sense of bewilderment when experiencing feelings that were never spoken about and that remained nameless. Such memories could be expected to produce a strong sense of being at risk and could also be linked to the occurrence of distressing images or dreams. Implicit memories may have a similar effect without being recognized as memories. Theoretically, these linked biases reinforce each other and maintain the problem (see also Chapter 2).

Borkovec's theory about the processes underlying worry in generalized anxiety disorder is also relevant (Borkovec, 1994; Borkovec, Alcaine, & Behar, 2004; Borkovec & Newman, 1998). Worry is seen as avoidance of the intense emotional arousal that occurs when anticipating contact with or having images of specific alarming situations.

The distress caused by worrying has been shown to be less than that caused by imagery (Butler, Wells, & Dewick, 1995; Wells & Papageorgiou, 1995). It is suggested that engaging in worry, or indeed in other cognitive activity, is a strategic response to anticipated threat that lowers arousal at the time, but which delays emotional processing. It is possible that a similar process is in operation when people avoid affect. Although there is no evidence that we know of to suggest that people who avoid affect are especially prone to worry, it is possible that the other strategies they use, such as distraction, focusing on physical sensations, disengagement, or dissociation, also have the (short-term) effect of reducing the intensity of emotional arousal. Avoidance of affect, in a similar way to worry, has the effect of cutting people off from (emotional) reality with the result that any emotional arousal remains threatening. The actual degree of threat cannot then be realistically judged or graded, and exaggerated or absolute ideas about emotions are reinforced; they cannot be disconfirmed while attempts to shut them out persist (Gross, 2007). As Borkovec often reminded us it is hard to develop the courage and skill to observe reality.

Hypotheses about the Development of Avoidance of Affect

The example of Douglas provided earlier in this chapter illustrates one type of experience described by patients who avoid affect and makes the assumption that this experience contributed to the development of the problem. However, it is important to bear in mind that there are at least four types of contributory factors of which experience is only one, as shown in Figure 7.1. Any or all of these factors may be relevant in an individual case.

When someone who avoids affect describes traumatic experiences or neglect in childhood, or when someone with a borderline personality disorder (BPD) becomes anxious, it may be worth considering whether this is a manifestation of the detached protector mode described by Young and colleagues (2003). When operating in this mode, which supposedly serves a self-protective function, someone may appear dispassionate and withdrawn, apparently cut off from the experience and the expression of emotions, and hypervigilant for the expression of emotion by others, including the therapist. In extreme cases "the patient shuts off all emotions, disconnects from others, and functions in an almost robotic manner" (pp. 307–308). This shutdown may be precipitated by fear of triggering early memories, for example, or by fear of "schema activation." Patients in distress tend to switch between modes as interpersonal situations in which they are involved change, and they may be able to learn to recognize these switches, and to take control of them once they have been able to form a stable, trusting relationship. This is therefore the first and most important task of the therapist working with someone who habitually avoids affect.

Undoubtedly, it is useful to attempt to understand the reasons that people have for avoiding affect, even if they are hard to elicit or to specify. Doing so collaboratively as part of the work of formulation also provides explicit and implicit messages (as described in Chapter 3, p. 69), for example, to the effect that it is possible to make sense of patients' experiences and difficulties; that they have good reasons for behaving as they do, and that these are understandable and changeable. These can help to reduce self-blame or feelings of shame that may otherwise accompany recognition of the problem.

Genetic or biological variation—for example, in speed of arousal or sensitivity to physiological changes.

Cultural factors—for example, the degree and type of emotional expression that is considered acceptable varies according to race, nationality, gender, age, religion, and so on.

Experience—for example, belonging to a family in which talking about feelings is not customary or acceptable. Painful or traumatic events that produce discomfort with feelings, such as humiliation, criticism, betrayal, rejection, bullying, cruelty, and so on. The experience of Type 2 trauma.

Posttraumatic stress disorder following specific (Type 1) trauma—This may be associated with symptoms of emotional numbing, but also with distressing intrusions and an exaggerated startle reaction, which may reinforce the fear of emotional arousal.

FIGURE 7.1. Causes and contributory factors to avoidance of affect.

Consequences

Understanding the consequences of avoidance of affect also contributes to formulation work. As in other anxiety disorders, maintenance cycles and patterns of behavior develop that prevent disconfirmation of fears and hence interfere with many aspects of life. Examples are shown in Figure 7.2.

People who spend much of their time withdrawing or protecting themselves from emotional arousal may predominantly see themselves as in retreat and therefore find it difficult to operate as effective agents of change in their own lives—their actions seem to be largely defensive. They may even be living in hypervigilant mode, constantly on the look out for threats. Although tension may be commonly experienced, relaxation is not always helpful, for example, when letting go brings distressing feelings with it and leads to increases in tension and anxiety. Altogether, the consequences of avoidance of affect feed into maintenance cycles and patterns of behavior that confirm existing thoughts, assumptions, and beliefs.

Consequences for therapy are clear. In extreme cases, giving voice to fears (verbalizing thoughts, expectations, predictions, assumptions, ideas, attitudes, etc.) about feel-

Interference with:

- Development of skills and confidence.
- Acquiring a vocabulary for talking about emotions.
- Self-discovery: the feeling of knowing oneself and of recognizing ones' likes, preferences, and values.
- Getting to know people, making friends, and communicating with others effectively.
- Developing intimate relationships.
- Organizing goal-directed behavior to meet functional needs; agency.
- Feeling motivated.

FIGURE 7.2. Some common consequences of avoidance of affect.

ings threatens to bring feelings with it and is also avoided. Negative automatic thoughts are especially hard to identify when the behaviors associated with them have been successful. For example, a patient who was adept at changing the topic if it threatened to become too personal and emotional did this frequently during therapy. However, the behavior was so automatic that she was unaware of doing it and unable, at first, to reflect on what triggered it (which of her thoughts or feelings were relevant, or which behavior of others was alarming to her, for instance). Stifling feelings of hostility, or of affection, reduces the risk of becoming "emotional," but also reduces the amount of information gathered during social interactions. So cognitions may be hard to access, and patients may deny having relevant thoughts, as if they have shut down the links between cognition and emotion. Being asked to "open up" is for them like entering unknown, and potentially dangerous territory. They give the impression of thinking "I can't go there" and "I mustn't let this happen," without being able to put such thoughts into words. Opening up emotionally in the relative safety of the therapy room can start the process of breaking maintenance cycles and disconfirming expectations—hence the need for therapists to assess carefully the current level of trust within the therapy relationship, and to remain alert for signs of distrust.

STRATEGIES FOR DEALING WITH AVOIDANCE OF AFFECT

The first priority is to develop an appropriate working relationship. This demands a high degree of sensitivity and an ability to adapt according to what is needed for different people. Showing warmth and empathy can be more alarming than encouraging for some. It helps to pay attention to what facilitates or impedes good communication, and to be alert to cultural differences. For example, a therapist was working with a person from a culture in which respect was highly valued, and respect was customarily shown through agreement and through efforts to conform and to please. The therapy was exceptionally difficult until the varying cultural expectations were brought up for discussion. Then it became clear that the more anxious this person felt, the more he tried to please, and the more tempted he was to hide the true extent of his difficulties and the details of his experience.

One of the many dilemmas therapists face is in balancing respect for privacy and sensitivity to distress on the one hand, with an attitude of acceptance and a belief in the need to face fears on the other. An understandable mistake commonly made by relatively inexperienced cognitive therapists is to focus too much on cognitions: to use the skills of Socratic questioning; to discuss, reason, challenge, and search for evidence instead of working to acknowledge, recognize, name, show, and talk about feelings, often working with the feelings that are present during therapy sessions. Standard cognitive methods are certainly useful, but the main criterion of success in using them is that they help people to *feel* better. If feelings are not present, then half the picture is missing. So the first aim is to plan exposure to feelings, which means accessing and helping someone to tolerate contact with aspects of experience that make that person feel most vulnerable. When this is done in a clear cognitive context, for example, using behavioral experiments to help people to reevaluate their thoughts, assumptions, and beliefs as has been described in detail by Butler and Surawy (2004), feelings and cognitions are more likely to change in synchrony. But to plan appropriate behavioral

> *The main aim is to help people to experience and to express their feelings:*
>
> - Listen for feelings, notice and identify them, then reflect them back.
> - Look for markers of emotional arousal (e.g., changes in posture, gaze, etc.).
> - Ask about physical sensations: "Where do you feel that?"
> - Ask about feelings: "What's that like?" Metaphors may be easier to use than words for feelings: "as if I'm about to burst" and "like stormy weather inside."
> - Make comments about them, such as, "You look sad when you say that," "Underneath you sound a bit hopeless," "That sounds like a real worry."
> - Return to them repeatedly.
> - Provide a language for talking about them: use emotion words and metaphors; model talking comfortably about feelings.
> - Show warmth, empathy, and other feelings as you normally would outside therapy, so as to increase familiarity with their expression in a safe context.

FIGURE 7.3. Basic strategies for eliciting feelings.

experiments one first has to develop an idea about what feelings mean to the person one is working with. Some of the basic strategies for eliciting feelings are shown in Figure 7.3.

Providing Information and Education

Providing information about feelings helps people to normalize their experience, and also to make sense of them. For example, our names for the main emotions are analogous to the names for primary colors. Most feelings, like most colors, are mixtures, and hence it is not surprising that they are difficult to name. Instead it may help to identify some of their elements: apprehension and irritation for instance; or frustration, fear, and hope. Another important point that many people find helpful comes from the gestalt view that feelings "reach for closure." An analogy with hunger is useful. Something provokes the feeling (the smell of newly baked bread, a long gap since the last meal), the feeling motivates the hungry person to do appropriate things (start cooking, go to a restaurant, buy a snack); then, provided the behavior is not interrupted, the hunger can be satisfied and will die away until something else provokes it and the cycle begins again. The hungry episode reaches closure provided the feeling is recognized and acted upon. The implication is that failing to recognize feelings and their motivating force, or trying to stop having or expressing them, will leave the feeling "open." This may explain the sense that some people have that allowing themselves to acknowledge their feelings will (at least initially) be overwhelming.

Sometimes it is necessary to start by developing a language for talking about feelings, even for people who do not suffer from alexithymia. A useful task is to collect a list of words for emotions, positive and negative, and then to search for observable instances of them, for example, when watching TV, or observing others in conversation. To ensure that the list is culturally appropriate to the person concerned the list can be made together, and others with whom the patient is in contact may be able to contribute. Some people need to practice recognizing signs of particular feelings in themselves and in others, and keeping a feeling diary may be helpful. There are many ways of doing this, one of which is provided in Figure 7.4. The aim of this diary was to help the person to recognize that his feelings were usually mixed, and that his thoughts and beliefs in a particular situation were linked to his feelings in intensity, and sometimes also in their complexity. Thinking about these links helped him to make sense of his feelings and to take them into account when deciding how to act.

> While cognitive therapists reject much of psychoanalytic theory, it is undeniable that many difficult, chronic patients seem actively to avoid looking at their deepest cognitions and emotions. Regardless of how this phenomenon is explained, therapists still must develop therapeutic strategies to deal with this avoidance, or else they will be continually stymied by personality disorder. (Young, 1990, p. 7)

Decatastrophizing

The main strategy of decatastrophizing is obvious, but explaining it can sound cruel: first, identify the predicted catastrophe, second, devise an experiment to allow or provoke feelings, and third, find out if the catastrophe occurs.

> In Tilly's family nobody spoke about feelings, and visible displays of emotion, whether positive or negative, were severely punished. As a small child she was

---

The person who used this diary had been confused by not being able to name his feelings, or to recognize their links with his thoughts and beliefs. The diary was constructed so as to help him to start to do this. He decided that the feelings listed should be randomly arranged, so as to remind him that mixtures could include unlikely combinations. He used the diary to work on specific, difficult situations.

Date:

Situation:

Emotion: 0–100

angry	anxious	apprehensive
sad	miserable	depressed
frightened	worried	irritated
pleased	frustrated	calm
frustrated	contented	happy
peaceful	bored	

Thinking: what was running through my mind (automatic thoughts)?

How much do I believe each of the thoughts (0–100)?

FIGURE 7.4. Example of a "feeling diary."

punished for laughing as well as for crying. As the oldest child in the family she was expected to keep her four younger siblings under control, and whenever they argued, fought, hurt themselves, or became boisterous she was punished as well as they. One of her problems as an adult was that her expressions of emotion were either minimal (a brief smile when something intensely pleased her) or maximal (exploding with anger after weeks of trying patiently to tolerate the dismissive and rude way in which she was treated by a neighbor). Her minimal expressions of emotion often went unnoticed by others and confirmed that something that was of great significance to her was of no importance to them. The maximal expressions were dismissed by others as "over the top" and then ignored. Both these responses confirmed her beliefs about the "badness" of showing her feelings: "My feelings don't matter, and shouldn't be counted."

For Tilly, decatastrophizing involved much preliminary work during which she learned to focus inwardly on bodily sensations. This helped to increase her awareness of feelings and her sensitivity to their early beginnings. At the next stage she learned to give the feelings a name and practiced trying to slow down her initial reactions. Eventually, when a friend said something appreciative, instead of finding a way of changing the topic, or laughing it off, she was able to pause, look at her, and try to say something that reflected the way she felt, however small, like "thank you." Of course friends do not offer compliments and show signs of appreciation just when they are needed for practicing homework assignments, and people who avoid affect need to practice expressing negative as well as positive feelings. So it is essential to explain the rationale for the overall strategy clearly, and it helps to role-play various ways of showing feelings—hence the general need to pay close attention to signs of emotional arousal during the session and to use these to identify feelings and to experiment with expressing them.

The work of decatastrophizing feelings is especially difficult for people who have become sensitized to feelings. For all of us, thinking or talking about a "hot" (or unprocessed) emotional event is likely to bring the feelings with it. When people avoid affect, a relatively innocuous event, or the memory of it during a therapy session, may trigger intense feelings that interfere with the ability to reflect on them. This experience should be normalized, and therapists can usefully introduce the notion of readiness here: asking patients if they are ready to talk about the event, helping them to accept the intense feelings, to name them and to allow them to come and to go. It may also be useful for patients to learn deep breathing exercises, or to develop the skills involved in relaxation or mindfulness meditation. These can assist the patient in accepting and learning about the experience of intense affect provided that they are not adopted as safety behaviors.

Paying Attention to Others

When awareness of the emotions of others is kept below the horizon this commonly results in increased self-awareness or self-focused attention, as has been described in the cognitive model of social phobia developed by Clark and Wells (1995). Support for this model of social phobia has been provided, for example, by research showing that people with social phobia are not as good as others at observing the facial expression of others (Mansell & Clark, 1999). Their ideas about the feelings of others (especially those with negative implications such as anger or disapproval) are thus based on inaccurate information and influenced by their own feelings and expectations. Conclusions are arrived at using guesswork combined with emotional reasoning.

> Sharon's feelings were easy to miss. She would say, with little expression: "I don't feel very well" or "I didn't do that quite right" when what she meant was that she felt utterly terrified and panicky, or that she had done something so badly that it would take months for others in the accounts department where she worked to put things right.

> Sharon, thought like this: "They are angry with me because I did something stupid" (even though others were not angry), and when she felt disapproved of she thought that others disapproved of her. She was, as such people usually are, completely unaware that her reasoning was "faulty" and believed that her impressions, based on her feelings, were correct. Helping her to focus externally instead, so as to pick up more accurate information about others, was difficult and took much practice. Her attention was repeatedly grabbed by internal thoughts and feelings, and she had to learn to expect this and to practice calmly redirecting her attention every time she noticed. In-session work helped her to do this. First, she practiced consciously switching her attention to specific (external) sights or sound, away from her internal experience, when requested to do so by the therapist. The aim at this stage was to learn to adopt an external focus at will and not to worry if her attention quickly wandered off again. The fact that attention constantly shifts was explained to her. Once she could do this she practiced switching attention during conversations with the therapist, so as to focus either internally, or on what was being said and on the interaction. This enabled her to observe the effects of different modes of attention on the quality of the interaction. (The method is described in detail in Butler, 1999b, pp. 145–160, and in these circumstances, attention training might also be used [Wells, 2000, pp. 139–147].) The work described above was combined with practice in methods of giving feedback as described next.

Using Feedback

The style of cognitive therapy offers excellent opportunities for practicing communicating about feelings, sometimes in situations that feel risky for the patient. The idea that both parties to the interaction need to keep in close touch with each other about "how they are doing" provides a framework for reflecting openly on feelings, during the work of the session and when reflecting on the process of therapy. Of course this can happen at any time, but asking patients for their reactions to the last session as they begin the new one, and for their comments on the current session as it ends, provides more formal opportunities that patients come to expect and can be asked to prepare for if they are regular parts of the agenda.

> Caro was depressed as well as anxious—predominantly about her ability to relate to other people, about their judgments of her, and her performance at work. In therapy sessions—as elsewhere—she found it hard to talk much. She warmed up slowly and then spoke more openly about the situations (present or past) that had distressed her. Having made contact with her feelings, she left each session feeling

much worse than when she had arrived. She found the experience of her feelings so distressing and the potential humiliation of showing them so great that she became openly ambivalent about continuing in therapy. Discussing the process of therapy and considering ways of adapting it so that she could feel more comfortable and make more use of it helped Caro to continue.

The first solution she tried was to take responsibility for bringing an important item for the agenda each time, and to give herself time to think ahead about what this should be. The item was then worked on first, with the result that her feelings became accessible earlier in the session, and there was time later on to reflect on the whole process. This involved considering how the session so far had felt for her, resolving as far as possible any remaining feelings of distress (partly through the process of mutual feedback), and dealing with her numerous reservations about bringing up painful material for discussion with another person. Honest feedback from the therapist included mention of feelings such as frustration about not being able to help more effectively at first, worry about sending her away feeling worse at the end of the session, relief at being able to understand Caro's feelings better, and feeling more hopeful about being able to work effectively together once the feelings were present. Caro had feared that talking about feelings would be like opening Pandora's box: All the demons inside would escape and successfully elude recapture, playing havoc with her ability to carry on her day-to-day life. Instead she found that she could deal with them slowly: one at a time, in a way that felt safe. The therapist in this case found that it was a mistake to have more than one major item on the agenda and changes came faster when the work was taken more slowly, and when Caro played a bigger part in initiating discussion.

Accepting Negative Feelings

Anger, disappointment, and other negative feelings can be especially difficult to talk about for patients who avoid affect. Much useful work can be done if therapists can facilitate the expression of doubts, reservations, and negative feelings about therapy and accept and validate these. Open discussion, accepting and understanding the reasons for these feelings, and attempting to resolve them provide ways of modeling how to go about finding a way forward. Sharon, whose feelings were initially so easy to miss when she said things like "I don't feel very good" had improved enormously when she said that she had been a bit uncomfortable at the end of the previous session. It took a large part of the session to discover that she had gone away furious and feeling put down because the therapist had dismissed one of her ideas about what to do for her next assignment. As far as the therapist remembered, all she did was elaborate on Sharon's suggestion so as to find a practical way forward. Talking it through de-catastrophized her fear of talking about anger and demonstrated that it was possible to reach a resolution and reduce her angry feelings without saying or doing anything dramatic or violent.

Making Use of Recordings

Sharon and her therapist had routinely tape-recorded all their sessions, and they were able to listen to the tape subsequently to check out what had actually been said, and to think again about what it meant, and what both parties thought it meant at the time. Such tape-recording is exceptionally useful when people avoid affect. Listening to the tape as a homework assignment can help give the patient a second chance to identify what he or she felt at the time (in private), and provide an opportunity to check out whether the feelings of another person (the therapist) have been accurately identified. Listening to the tape can also help the therapist to identify small signs of emotion, or to elaborate on and make distinctions between feelings that the patient may have showed but that were hard to express or to name at the time. Video-recordings can potentially provide even more useful information, if the equipment is available and the patient is willing to make them and watch them.

Using Metaphor

Talking about abstract concepts such as feelings is hard to do without using metaphors. Indeed metaphors provide us with precise and informative descriptions of another person's emotional state ("I feel torn apart" and "... tied up in knots"). So we should pay careful attention to the metaphors our patients use to describe their feelings and see whether we can find a way of using these metaphors, and others too, to help the process of therapy along. Common metaphors used by people who avoid affect include being well defended, or walled-up; living in a prison; being cut off from others; feeling as if there is a pane of glass between you and them; and being frozen or even dead inside. Contrasting metaphors for example involve coming alive again, throwing open the windows, lifting the lid of the box, or making a window so that the light can shine into the prison. These can be extremely useful when someone is starting to talk more about her or his feelings. It is as if the metaphor enables people to initiate exposure to feelings and provides a step on the (somewhat bumpy) road to talking about them more freely as well as experiencing them more fully—and the process can also feel more lighthearted. Asking what the person wants to do when she feels like that (e.g., to run away, to cry, to seek comfort, to fight back) can also initiate the process of making more functional use of feelings. It contributes to the development of a sense of agency and creates direct links with behavioral work, which can then provide experience of the value of feelings, of the importance of expressing them, and of the possibility of behaving in ways that help to resolve them.

Words are not the only ways of representing and expressing feelings of course. They can be expressed through any creative medium such as writing, drawing, music, and movement or dance, through making something, or by taking action, and so on. The ways of expressing and using compassionate imagery to counteract self-criticism and self-denigration described by Gilbert (e.g., 2005a) are especially useful for providing a sense of comfort that can contribute to the recognition of painful feelings and for resolution of distress (for a detailed example of how to do this see Lee, 2005). The underlying messages are that accepting and expressing feelings, although it can make people feel vulnerable, is important and necessary, and that feelings can be represented in numerous ways. Patients should be encouraged to use any ways they feel comfortable with. Two unusual examples from clinical practice include making small clay figures (models of attentive, kind people as a reminder that others can accept bad feelings), and making a cube-shaped lavender bag. Squeezing this to release the scent helped the person who made it to ground herself in the present when she felt at risk of going blank or dissociating, and its edges and corners reminded her that painful "hard" stuff could be softened if she could accept and keep in touch with it. These two examples demonstrate an originality and creativity that obviously could not be directed by the therapist, so it is important to think about the part played by the therapist in releasing, or encouraging, this kind of creativity. One possibility is that being explicit about the importance of feelings, and accepting of different ways of expressing them, perhaps illustrated by the use of metaphor, provides valuable setting conditions. Then sometimes all that is needed is to ask people to think about how they would like to express their feelings, reminding them that there are numerous possibilities, and perhaps suggesting that they explore methods that seem natural to them, such as drawing pictures for people who use a lot of imagery, using poetry or music for people more inclined in those directions.

Implicit Memory: A Way of Making Sense

All his adult life Jerry had kept moving from one place to another. He was tempted to move on again whenever his relationships with the people around him threatened to become more open and friendly. He was desperately lonely and had attended an assertiveness class to develop his social confidence but was unable to do the practical exercises that were suggested. In conversation generally he said his mind went blank, and when assessed for treatment he appeared intermittently distracted and disconnected. He described his loneliness and inability to achieve his goals but was unable to provide details of specific situations or to describe how they made him feel. He kept asking the therapist to repeat the question and explained that he felt unreal much of the time, "as if living behind a pane of glass."

Jerry's symptoms of derealization were exacerbated by the process of therapy, and his reactions to these symptoms provided the original clue that helped the therapist to find out what was happening.

It gradually became clear that Jerry had been physically abused throughout his childhood and had also been assaulted on his way home from school when he was age 13 by a gang of teenagers. He used to enjoy working in his garden until one day intense fear and a feeling of impending panic broke through his calmness. He was unable to explain this event until asked how it might link up with his past. Then he said that it made him think of the hillside on the day of his assault. The light was falling on the ground around him in a similar way, and it was the same time of year. The ground smelled the same. His implicit memory of this event (memory without awareness that it was a memory) had triggered the emotional response that he had been at such pains to avoid. This demonstration of emotional links between past and present enabled him to start letting his guard down, and talking in more detail about his feelings about his childhood experiences, and about his current fear that accessing feelings would make him vulnerable to increasingly intense and uncontrollable emotions that "would not change anything."

Reducing the Use of Safety-Seeking Behaviors

People who avoid affect use safety-seeking behaviors to reduce the likelihood of talking about feelings, and to lower the chances of provoking unwanted expressions of feeling in others. Common safety-seeking behaviors include distraction, joking, intellectualizing, changing the topic, and disengaging, but there are many others also. When self-protection has high priority even the patient may not be aware of habitual ways of responding to situations that feel threatening, for instance, if voices are raised, or if wanting to join a group of others who suddenly start laughing, or when closer acquaintance leads (potentially) to greater degrees of intimacy.

Behavioral experiments, constructed in the ways described in Chapter 6 (pp. 113–116) are needed to test all relevant levels of cognition, and detailed examples can be found in Butler and Surawy (2004). In this context it is useful to add a reminder of the sandwich principle described in Chapter 3 (pp. 64–67). Difficult formulation work, and practical work, can be held together by using this principle. It is especially useful when the precise context within which distress arises varies, as it is highly likely to do when avoidance of affect is an issue, as different situations will elicit different feelings. In outline, the principle suggests that consistency in the work can be provided by thinking in terms of both slices of bread in the sandwich: beliefs and behaviors. For example, behavioral experiments, such as those involved in letting your feelings show, should be constructed with an underlying belief in mind, such as the belief that displays of emotion will be punished. Then the outcome of the experiment can be evaluated in relation to the belief irrespective of the particular emotion expressed.

This method was used to help Jerry reconsider his belief that displays of feelings turn other people against you. First his therapist explained to him more about emotions as described above (p. 143), and then together they clarified specific, testable predictions. The work was started using in-session material because this was immediately accessible, less threatening or risky for Jerry, and otherwise his self-protective, avoidant habits might have got in the way. One of his first predictions was, "If I let my feelings show we won't be able to do any proper work, and you will get irritated with me." They decided that the therapist would take the lead and ask Jerry, whenever he started to withdraw, or seemed emotionally detached from the material being discussed, to pay attention to his bodily sensations, describe them, try to amplify them, and to give them a name. Reactions to doing this were discussed at length, paying attention to Jerry's and the therapist's point of view, and thinking about how talking about feelings affected the work of the session and about Jerry's belief that showing feelings would turn people against him. The predictions subsequently tested were graduated and always specific, for example: "If I talk about feeling lonely I will only feel worse" and "If I tell my house mates that I am tired of taking responsibility for dealing with the trash and ask them to share the work they will blow up at me," and so on. As Jerry's avoidance of affect decreased he became more accepting of his own, and of others', feelings; he started to become curious about the effects of showing (relatively innocuous) feelings and became less rigid in his attempts to keep them hidden.

PITFALLS AND DIFFICULTIES

A number of difficulties commonly arise when working with people who avoid affect. On the assumption that forewarned is forearmed, the main ones are identified in the lists below. Some of these were already mentioned above and are listed here for quick reference. Others follow from the arguments presented above. They are organized into two main categories: those primarily affecting the therapist and those primarily affecting the patient, while recognizing that, whatever the source of the difficulty, it is likely to affect both parties through the interaction between them.

Those Primarily Affecting the Therapist

- Colluding with avoidance. It is easy to collude with someone who is amusing, or interesting, or who has become especially skilled at diverting attention from feelings. It is also easy when feelings are intense and distressing, or when a therapist is not comfortable with a particular feeling (e.g., hostility or anger).
- Focusing too much on cognitions (or on behavior).
- Difficulty identifying cognitions, owing to the absence of observable affect shifts.
- The absence of emotional expression can make the patient appear distant, cut off, disconnected from others, and even "unreachable."
- Mistaking compliance, co-operation, and other ways of pleasing the therapist for "health" or recovery.
- Offering too much, or inappropriate, self-disclosure.
- Feeling disconnected from, and unable to relate well to a patient.

Those Primarily Affecting the Patient

- Talking about feelings rather than expressing them.
- Experiencing feelings in an "all or nothing" way: being unable to modulate the experience of affect.
- Withdrawing, or shutting down, in response to present feelings.
- Forgetting, detaching, or going blank: being unable to make contact with what feelings were like, or what it was like to have them in the past.
- Feeling worse as the avoidance and safety-seeking behaviors are reduced, within or across sessions.
- Ambivalence about engaging in treatment.
- Uncertainty about what others are feeling (this can affect the therapist as well as the patient).
- Uncertainties about social and cultural conventions, and about the appropriateness of expressing emotions in specific situations.

CONCLUSION

Those who avoid affect do so for their own good reasons. They may avoid experiencing, expressing, or provoking their own feelings, or avoid the experience and the expression of feelings in others, or they may avoid in both ways. Their reasons, at one level, are based on the sense that feelings are risky, threatening, or dangerous and contact with them therefore makes them vulnerable. Common hypotheses, of value in formulation work, suggest that people learn to avoid affect because doing so was useful at an early (earlier) stage of development. Cutting oneself off from feelings, or developing a habit of distancing oneself from them, may have reduced suffering and distress. However, impoverished emotional experience makes it hard to know what you want and hard to meet your own needs (for affiliation, comfort, protection, companionship, caring, etc.). It makes it hard to develop a stable and consistent sense of who you are—of the individuality that is expressed in likes and dislikes, and in characteristic ways of setting about meeting personal goals.

The therapy relationship is therefore one of the most potent tools for recognizing the problem in action and for developing ways of overcoming it. However this is only the beginning, and once the world of feelings has started to open up, subsequent cognitive work helping people to question and find alternatives to their ideas about emotion, and behavioral work, of the kind described in more detail in the previous chapter, can then be used to great advantage. Experiments involving feelings, for example, trying out different ways of expressing them, in different contexts is likely to have the added advantage that it assists the patient in making more functional and reinforcing connections and links with others. Those experiential techniques that focus on the experience and expression of affect in the therapy room are generally too alarming for these people to use at first. However, when they are more comfortable with feelings they may also benefit more from these and become better situated to use their feelings to meet their own needs.

EIGHT

Low Self-Esteem

In our first chapter, we highlighted the essential themes and associated cognitive and behavioral maintenance processes that define different anxiety disorders and briefly outlined contemporary treatment protocols designed to target these with maximum efficiency by addressing issues and processes specific to each disorder. We also noted that individual anxiety disorders are frequently comorbid not only with other anxiety disorders, but also with a range of other difficulties. In particular, readers scanning Chapter 1 will discover that low self-esteem can be implicated in the development and persistence of anxiety disorders right across the spectrum. This can raise problems for the clinician: problems in understanding how the different facets of the patient's difficulties interrelate, and problems in determining how to devise a coherent, efficient treatment program that addresses not just the anxiety, but also other elements as well.

Background low self-esteem can be problematic in a number of ways. It may produce a confusing picture where patients present with anxiety alongside significant depression, and it is hard to say which came first, which is the more important, and which should be the initial treatment priority. Sometimes the picture is even more complicated: A central negative sense of self may be at the root of a wide range of problems, as was the case with Gordon and Leo whose cases are described below. Sometimes patients' efforts to change are sabotaged by habitual self-critical thinking and hopelessness, they become depressed when treatment does not progress according to plan, or indeed they may view working on their anxieties as trivial in comparison to their global negative sense of self. And even those whose anxiety is successfully treated using one of the specific treatment protocols outlined in Chapter 1 may remain vulnerable to relapse if underlying low self-esteem is left untouched. A possible solution, when therapists realize that low self-esteem is a generalized background problem, is to use a conceptual framework that acknowledges its central significance and understands anxiety, depression, and so on in relation to it.

The cognitive model of low self-esteem that is the focus of this chapter provides just such a framework. It offers a specific, transdiagnostic framework within which to understand the origins and development of patients' problems, and to investigate how they interlink in the present day. The chapter shows how fundamental issues of identity and self-worth, often central to the distress of patients who are anxious, can be effectively treated using the systematic and practical focus of cognitive therapy. The model (Fennell, 1997) forms the basis for an integrated program of interventions deriving from established evidence-based protocols for specific emotional disorders and from cognitive approaches to working with enduring negative beliefs about the self (e.g., Beck et al., 2004; Young et al., 2003). Unlike the specific treatment protocols that were our starting point, this approach is transdiagnostically applicable because it addresses common cognitive and behavioral processes that occur across a range of emotional disorders, and indeed personality patterns. In particular, it offers a means of understanding the intimate relationship that can link comorbid anxiety and depression.

A COGNITIVE PERSPECTIVE

The term "low self-esteem" refers to a sense of lacking value or worth, *as a person*, of weighing oneself in the balance and finding oneself wanting. Low self-esteem reflects broad negative beliefs about the self (schemas or core beliefs) that generally derive from experience (often, but not necessarily, early in life) and that, once established, influence how people interpret what happens to them on a day-to-day basis, their emotional state, and what they do. Thus low self-esteem can be viewed as a self-maintaining process in which enduring negative perspectives shape current thoughts, emotions, and behaviors, and these in turn feed back into and strengthen the negative sense of self. This reciprocal feedback loop, between immediate processing and more enduring cognitive structures, can result in a system that is extremely robust, and indeed resistant to change.

THE RELATIONSHIP BETWEEN ANXIETY AND LOW SELF-ESTEEM

People who are anxious often make negative statements about themselves that might be taken to reflect enduring low self-esteem (e.g., "I'm useless," "I'm pathetic," "I'm unattractive," "I'm no good"). However, the relationship between negative self-statements and presenting problems can vary (Fennell, 1997). They might reflect a negative sense of self that is primarily an aspect of the presenting problem, a consequence of it, or a vulnerability factor that predisposes people to a range of different problems. And these different roles can interact. For example, a long-standing negative sense of self usually intensifies in response to depressed mood and may be strengthened by the onset of clinical anxiety for which there seems to be no solution.

Low Self-Esteem as an Aspect of Presenting Problems

In some cases, a negative perspective on the self may be primarily an aspect of an immediate problem. Classically, this is the case with depression, where negative thoughts about the self are seen as central to the phenomenology (Beck et al., 1979, p. 11). As depression lifts (whether via psychological treatment interventions, medication, or the simple passage of time) so a balanced sense of self often returns, without a need to address self-esteem in its own right. This is an important consideration, given the high frequency with which anxiety is comorbid with depression in routine clinical practice. We should be wary of assuming that, for patients who are significantly depressed when they enter therapy, treatment will necessarily be extended by a need to work at length on enduring negative beliefs about the self, or that we should head straight for schema-focused cognitive therapy (cf. James, 2001). This may indeed turn out to be the case—but it may not.

Low Self-Esteem as a Consequence of Presenting Problems

In other cases, the negative sense of self is primarily a consequence of the limitations placed on a person's life by anxiety itself. Chronic and disabling anxiety can produce a pervasive drop in self-confidence and self-esteem. So, for example, long-standing ago-raphobia can undermine a person's sense of self-efficacy. Many years of generalized anxiety disorder (GAD) can result in demoralization and loss of confidence (Butler & Anastasiades, 1988). Even specific phobias can feed into a negative sense of self. The fact of having the phobia at all can be seen as a sign of weakness or inadequacy ("This is ridiculous. What would people think if they knew?"), as can hopelessness about the possibility of change ("This is me. I'm stuck with this"). More dramatically, posttrau-matic stress disorder (PTSD) can result in a "shattering" of previous positive beliefs about the self (Janoff-Bulman, 1992) and radical reappraisals of personal competence or worth, sometimes at a relatively late stage in life (see pp. 158–159). Again, in many of these cases, working effectively with the anxiety disorder may well restore a balanced sense of self without the need specifically to target self-esteem.

Low Self-Esteem as a Vulnerability Factor for Presenting Problems

Finally, a negative sense of self may act as a vulnerability factor predisposing patients to a range of anxiety disorders. Indeed, it may form the nexus for a constellation of diverse problems, including anxiety, which can initially be confusing to therapist and patient. The case illustrated in Figure 8.1, Gordon, did not meet formal diagnostic crite-ria for any specific anxiety disorder, and thus provides an example of someone to whom no established treatment protocol was readily applicable. The "vicious flower" shown in Figure 8.1 provided a relatively straightforward way of encapsulating his case formulation (see Chapter 4, pp. 78–80, for details on how to draw up "vicious flowers"). It was drawn up with Gordon once early sessions had clarified the diversity and complexity of his problems. For him, multiple anxieties (especially centered on work, relationships and emotional control) coexisted with emotional lability, bouts of heavy drinking, interpersonal difficulties, and depression. His central sense of self ("I am unacceptable") was placed at the center of the "flower," and the "petals" illustrate dysfunctional assumptions that governed his emotional and behavioral responses in everyday situations. The arrows show how "I am unacceptable" and a range of assumptions (and associated strategies) reciprocally reinforce one another. A more-or-less constant high level of anxiety was central to Gordon's problems, and his main rea-son for seeking help. It fueled his difficulties with others in that his responses to situa-tions relevant to his network of assumptions produced a range of unhelpful responses,

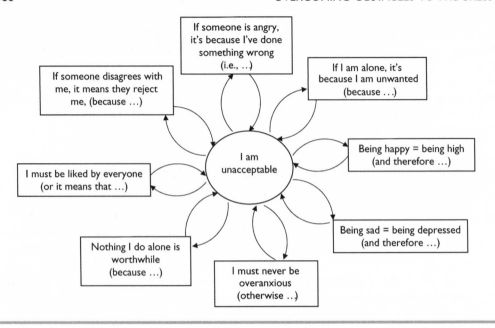

FIGURE 8.1. Low self-esteem as a central root for diverse problems.

ranging from alcohol consumption designed to help him to relax in social situations to fierce attempts to keep his emotional state within what he considered the "normal" range that made it hard for him to respond with warmth and spontaneity or to show distress.

How can we make sense of such complicated pictures, where even relatively straightforward, diagnosable anxiety disorders may turn out to be just one stone in a complex mosaic of problems and concerns? As implied by Figure 8.1, a focus on low self-esteem can provide just such a framework because it allows us to understand how different elements fit together and to investigate whether (as in this case) diverse difficulties might spring from a common source.

A COGNITIVE MODEL OF LOW SELF-ESTEEM

A cognitive model of low self-esteem is illustrated in the flowchart in Figure 8.2. It offers a framework for making sense of multiple anxieties and other comorbid difficulties, and thus a basis for an integrated, coherent treatment approach.

The model suggests that, on the basis of experience, people reach conclusions about themselves that are here termed the "bottom line." This means central negative beliefs about the self, which could be summarized in the form of sentences beginning "I am. . . . " "Experience" may include relationships with primary caregivers, relationships with others (e.g., siblings, the extended family, peers, and teachers), life circumstances (e.g., socioeconomic status, material conditions), events (e.g., trauma, bereavement, frequent moves), and broader sociopolitical influences such as religious and cultural context (e.g., being a member of a religious group with a punitive moral frame-

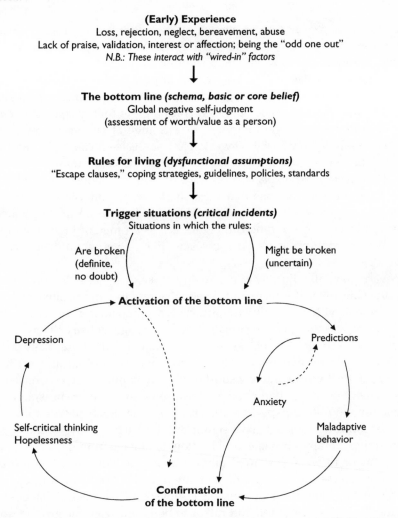

(Early) Experience
Loss, rejection, neglect, bereavement, abuse
Lack of praise, validation, interest or affection; being the "odd one out"
N.B.: These interact with "wired-in" factors

↓

The bottom line *(schema, basic or core belief)*
Global negative self-judgment
(assessment of worth/value as a person)

↓

Rules for living *(dysfunctional assumptions)*
"Escape clauses," coping strategies, guidelines, policies, standards

↓

Trigger situations *(critical incidents)*
Situations in which the rules:

Are broken
(definite,
no doubt)

Might be broken
(uncertain)

Activation of the bottom line

Depression

Predictions

Anxiety

Self-critical thinking
Hopelessness

Maladaptive
behavior

**Confirmation
of the bottom line**

FIGURE 8.2. A cognitive model of low self-esteem. Based on Fennell (1997).

work, being a member of a group that attracts hostility from a larger host culture, or being caught in a clash between two cultures, as can be the experience of second generation migrants).

Experience may interact with "wired-in factors" present from birth or shortly thereafter (such as temperament, physical appearance, physical or mental disability) in such a way as to influence sense of self from an early age. So, for example, a patient who later developed social phobia was born with nearsightedness (a "wired-in factor") that meant that she had to wear thick glasses throughout her childhood. She became a target for teasing, not only at school but also from her siblings. This led to a sense of inadequacy, and to an enduring mistrust of others' good intentions toward her.

Where the bottom line is negative, the consequence is low self-esteem. This forms fertile soil in which anxiety can grow. The intensity and consistency of the bottom line will vary from person to person, depending on, for example, whether experience has also provided access to alternative, more positive perspectives. So low self-esteem can be thought of as falling on a continuum (Fennell, 1998, 2004) in relation to how intense and consistent it is, how much impact it has on the person's life, and how easy (or difficult) it is to change. In some cases, where alternative perspectives are available, the negative sense of self emerges only in highly specific circumstances, such as an examination, a job interview, or a change of circumstances requiring the formation of a whole new social network. Here self-esteem can be thought of as fragile, rather than consistently low. At the far end of the continuum, however, we find people whose negative perspective on the self is more or less constantly activated, and who have little or no sense that there might be any alternative, kinder perspective. Here the degree of distress and disability is likely to be much greater, and the person may report long-standing difficulties across a range of life situations, and significant interpersonal problems. Such cases are likely to attract a diagnosis of personality disorder.

This variation will naturally affect treatment (Fennell, 2004). People with relatively situation-specific low self-esteem and potential access to more positive alternatives are likely to present with relatively straightforward encapsulated problems, to find the cognitive therapy rationale congenial, and to engage constructively in treatment (including independent self-help assignments). Equally, they are likely to be able to rapidly form collaborative relationships with their therapists, and difficulties and issues between the two are unlikely substantially to hinder progress. Consequently, it is easier for them to change than people whose sense of worthlessness, unlovability, or inadequacy is the only perspective available to them. Such people may well report chronic, generalized problems, have significant doubts about the validity or relevance of the cognitive therapy rationale, and be slow to engage in therapy. They may find it hard to focus or to work systematically on their problems, and therapy is likely to include numerous setbacks, times of stagnation, and a need to work repeatedly with the therapeutic relationship. Here the task is, not so much to reestablish or strengthen a preexisting positive sense of self, but rather to build one from the ground up. Thus the task of therapist and patient is harder, and therapy is likely to be more drawn out. For the therapist, this work requires patience, persistence, ingenuity, and well-developed interpersonal skills.

Late Onset of Low Self-Esteem

The above suggests that low self-esteem arises from early experience. However, this need not be the case. Doubts about oneself and anxieties about relationships often first appear in adolescence or early adulthood, when the person is facing numerous changes and challenges. Negative experiences with others at this stage (e.g., being bullied, ostracized, ridiculed, or rejected) can have a lasting impact on a young person's sense of self. Even much later in life, a preexisting, genuinely positive bottom line can be damaged or even radically undermined by experience, most dramatically in the case of exposure to traumatic events and subsequent PTSD. Paradoxically, people who with good reason value themselves for their strength, competence, and ability to cope may be particularly vulnerable here. Clinical experience suggests that such people are common in the armed forces and the emergency services, where their courage and resourcefulness are true assets. However, if during a traumatic event they find themselves behaving in ways that they repudiate (for instance, failing to save a comrade in a burning house), they may begin to doubt themselves. When subsequently they are unable readily to control posttraumatic symptoms using their usual, active coping strategies, this too may prompt a reevaluation of how they see themselves ("I thought I was strong. But now I can't manage my feelings, pull myself together, and get back to normal. I must have been wrong."). For such people, coming for therapy in itself may be seen as an admission of unacceptable weakness. This means that the therapist will need to proceed with caution, not only emphasizing that posttraumatic symptomatology is a normal human response to extreme events, but also suggesting that therapy is not a means of undermining old coping strategies, but rather an opportunity to add extra strings to the patient's bow—to enhance her or his already considerable competence in the face of stress.

Equally, there may be no need here to work extensively on creating and strengthening a positive sense of self. Rather, the most helpful focus may be on introducing greater flexibility into how positive qualities are defined and the over-stringent demands the patient places upon him- or herself, that is, work at the level of dysfunctional assumptions, or what the model calls "rules for living" (see below). So for example, a patient who before the onset of PTSD had always seen himself as "strong" took this to mean that he must *always* be able to control his mind and emotions, and that he should *never* need help in problem solving. Patient and therapist moved toward a more helpful alternative that acknowledged human beings' universal fallibility (i.e., that it is not possible to be superhuman), and that being strong can include having powerful emotions and unexpected thoughts, and knowing when asking for help is the wisest thing to do. Work on assumptions may also be centrally important where the sense of self has been compromised by less dramatic changes in life circumstances—for example, the onset of ageing in a person who has always prided herself on her youthful good looks, or loss of employment for a person whose sense of self-worth is predicated on being a good provider for others.

THE ROLE OF RULES FOR LIVING

To negotiate their way through life, given the apparent truth of the bottom line, people develop strategies encapsulated in "rules for living" (dysfunctional conditional assumptions, in cognitive therapy terms) that allow them to feel reasonably good about themselves, so long as the terms of the rules are met. Such rules are shaped by family and cultural norms (e.g., the protestant work ethic, gender stereotypes). They determine what the person must do or be to succeed in life, make and keep satisfying relationships, be happy, and so forth. However, they are frequently rigid and extreme, so that the effort of behaving in accordance with them is considerable, and there is a strong likelihood that at some point in people's life their terms will not be met. The requirements for "strength" outlined above in the section on late onset of low self-esteem would be an example. Another would be an absolute demand for perfectionism, as opposed to taking pleasure in and appreciating the value of doing things well.

HOW THE BOTTOM LINE IS TRIGGERED

If situations arise in which the rules *have definitely been broken*, or in which they *might be broken*, the bottom line is activated.

When the rules *have definitely been broken* (there is no doubt), the response is likely to be depressed in nature and is illustrated by the long dotted line running from "Activation" to "Confirmation" in the vicious circle at the bottom of Figure 8.2. Breaking the rule seems to confirm the truth of the bottom line, leading to self-critical ruminations and a sense of hopelessness ("This is me, so how can I ever change?"). Such negative thinking is likely then to feed into depressed mood, which may be transitory, but could intensify into the beginning of a clinical depression that might require treatment in its own right.

HOW LOW SELF-ESTEEM IS MAINTAINED

When the rules *might be broken* (i.e., there is an element of doubt), a different reaction follows, that leads us straight into the heart of anxiety. Activation of the bottom line here leads to the kind of negative predictions we know to be characteristic of anxiety, a complementary overestimation of the likelihood and magnitude of negative outcomes, and underestimation of internal or external resources by which catastrophe might be managed (the anxiety equation, Chapter 2, p. 30). Anxiety follows, and its symptoms or its very presence may in turn become a focus for further predictions (e.g., "I'm about to lose it"). This feedback process is illustrated by the short dotted line between "Predictions" and "Anxiety" on the righthand side of the vicious circle at the bottom of Figure 8.2. At the same time, a range of maladaptive behaviors come into play:

1. The situation in which the rule might be broken is avoided outright.
2. The person enters the situation but engages in safety-seeking behaviors that prevent her from discovering whether her predictions are correct and may even make the situation worse. For example, someone might avoid speaking openly about herself to not be rejected, but in fact appear cold and secretive, thus producing in others the withdrawal she fears—which she then believes confirms what she first thought. Safety-seeking behaviors can be extensively elaborated, for example, creating a false persona to hide what is seen as an unattractive self, adopting an aggressive stance to cover perceived weakness, and misuse of prescribed or street drugs.
3. Anxiety leads to genuine inhibitions in performance (such as clumsiness or going blank) that the person then interprets as further evidence of inadequacy, rather than understanding them as understandable consequences of high arousal.
4. All goes well. But far from being encouraged by this to reevaluate the bottom line, the person ignores the new information, discounts it, distorts the meaning of it (e.g., "Ah, but if I hadn't kept a very tight rein on my emotions, I *would* have fallen apart"), or decides that it is an exception to the rule (Padesky, 1994).

Thus the system more or less guarantees that, whatever happens, the bottom line will seem to have been confirmed. The sense of confirmation may take the form of explicit thoughts (e.g., "There you are, I really *am* boring"), or it might be an image, or a wordless felt sense, or even a change in the body (e.g., a heaviness or a sinking in the gut). However it is experienced, it moves the person across to the lefthand side of the maintenance cycle, away from anxiety and into the territory of depression. Once mood drops, the circle closes: Depression supports continued activation of negative thinking about the self and reinforces anticipation of negative outcomes.

Patients with low self-esteem sometimes oscillate between anxious and depressed maintenance processes (Fennell, 2006a). Thus a person might enter treatment while seriously depressed and withdrawn. As mood improves, returning to activities and relationships that have been avoided while depressed can trigger doubts and anxiety, perhaps sufficiently strong to stimulate withdrawal—and a return to depression. The model helps us to understand how these two states of mind (anxiety and depression) can interact, and to find a possible common foundation in low self-esteem.

TREATING COMORBID ANXIETY AND DEPRESSION: A CASE EXAMPLE

The cognitive model of low self-esteem can help to make sense of comorbidity and offers a useful option for understanding and working with some of the complex anxiety cases we discussed in Chapter 3. We use a case example (a patient who followed the anxious route) to illustrate this.

Presenting Problems at Referral

Leo was referred for treatment by his family doctor because he was becoming increasingly crippled by social phobia. The doctor was concerned that Leo would be unable to continue his studies and that this might have serious consequences for his future. In addition, she was aware that he was becoming more and more depressed and hopeless about the possibility of change, and worried that his occasional suicidal thoughts might develop into something more dangerous.

Leo had been told about cognitive therapy by another student who had found it helpful and specifically requested it because he liked its practicality and thought it made sense. He met diagnostic criteria for social phobia (generalized enough also to meet criteria for avoidant personality disorder), and this was identified as his main problem at the time of referral. Leo was pursuing a degree in media studies at a local university and had been finding it increasingly difficult to pursue his studies because of his fear of making a fool of himself if he spoke up in teaching sessions, and his sense that if he showed his work it would be ridiculed by staff and fellow students. Coming to the university was Leo's first experience of living away from home, and he said that he was finding the need to manage living independently, and especially to make new friends and perhaps find a girlfriend, highly anxiety provoking. He was afraid that other people would think him boring, stupid, and immature. He had become isolated and, although he did not meet criteria for major depressive episode, his mood was low. As his doctor noted, there were times when he wondered about suicide—it was hard to see any other way out of his difficulties.

Initial Therapy Sessions

Leo agreed that his social anxiety was a priority. Accordingly, treatment began by using the Clark and Wells (1995) model of social phobia as a framework for conceptualizing his difficulties (see Chapter 1, pp. 12–14). In early sessions, he and his therapist identified unhelpful social safety-seeking behaviors (see "Maintenance Processes" below) and discovered the impact of using or dropping them in a sequence of behavioral experiments within and between sessions. As described in Chapter 6, these were closely interwoven with cognitive work. For example, Leo learned how to question the validity of his anxious expectations as a prelude to testing them in action, to be aware of positive and negative aspects of social encounters instead of focusing only on what went wrong, and to spot and counter the biases in his "postmortems." Therapy appeared to be progressing well.

A Conundrum Emerges

After six sessions, however, Leo told his therapist that, in a seminar, he had had a panic attack. And this was not the first—in fact he had been having one or two panics every week for some while. Initially it appeared that the panic attacks were simply swift peaks of social anxiety, but closer inspection revealed a different picture. When he panicked, Leo hyperventilated and, as is often the case, became light-headed and dizzy. It turned out that his main fear was that he would pass out, and never come round again—he would die. This conviction dated from two early experiences of medical procedures (an injection and blood being taken) when he had indeed passed out and had been convinced at the time that he was dying. Now he was worrying that he would panic again, with fatal consequences.

So suddenly we have two extra diagnoses: panic disorder and blood injury phobia. And once again, this was not the full story. It emerged that Leo was not only afraid of dying when he panicked, he was also concerned about his health in a more general sense. He was alert to any changes in his physical condition and tended to assume that aches and pains or minor illnesses heralded the onset of something serious. He had been to his family doctor with "skin cancer" and "multiple sclerosis," and when reassured that his symptoms were benign felt too embarrassed to push for further investigations, but nonetheless remained unconvinced. He tended to explore his body for sinister signs, and to become preoccupied with anything he found. In fact, he said that the point was approaching where he could worry about anything and everything, and if there was nothing to worry about, then he would go and find something. Because he felt increasingly uncertain and out of control, he had begun attempting to take control of his life—tidying, cleaning, checking his work repeatedly for errors.

How could we make sense of this increasingly complex and confusing picture?

How Leo's Problems Developed (Figure 8.3)

Early Experience

Leo was the third of three brothers. At home, he always had the sense of being left behind. He would try to join in the games and conversations of his older brothers, but

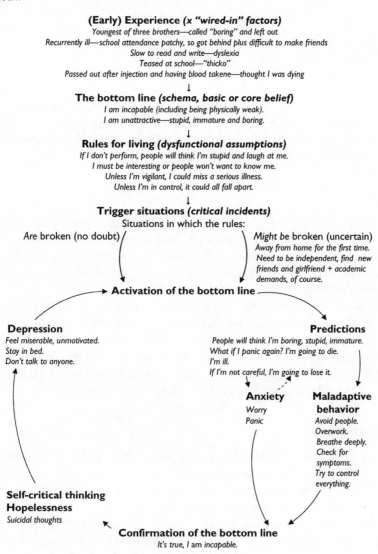

(Early) Experience *(x "wired-in" factors)*
Youngest of three brothers—called "boring" and left out
Recurrently ill—school attendance patchy, so got behind plus difficult to make friends
Slow to read and write—dyslexia
Teased at school—"thicko"
Passed out after injection and having blood takene—thought I was dying

↓

The bottom line *(schema, basic or core belief)*
I am incapable (including being physically weak).
I am unattractive—stupid, immature and boring.

↓

Rules for living *(dysfunctional assumptions)*
If I don't perform, people will think I'm stupid and laugh at me.
I must be interesting or people won't want to know me.
Unless I'm vigilant, I could miss a serious illness.
Unless I'm in control, it could all fall apart.

↓

Trigger situations *(critical incidents)*
Situations in which the rules:

Are broken (no doubt)   Might be broken (uncertain)
Away from home for the first time.
Need to be independent, find new
friends and girlfriend + academic
demands, of course.

Activation of the bottom line

Depression   **Predictions**
Feel miserable, unmotivated.   *People will think I'm boring, stupid, immature.*
Stay in bed.   *What if I panic again? I'm going to die.*
Don't talk to anyone.   *I'm ill.*
                                      If I'm not careful, I'm going to lose it.

                              Anxiety   **Maladaptive**
                              Worry   **behavior**
                              Panic   *Avoid people.*
                                                 Overwork.
                                                 Breathe deeply.
                                                 Check for
                                                 symptoms.
                                                 Try to control
Self-critical thinking   *everything.*
Hopelessness
Suicidal thoughts

                    Confirmation of the bottom line
                        It's true, I am incapable.

FIGURE 8.3. Cognitive model of low self-esteem: Clinical example (Leo).

their response all too often was to say "bo-ring" in a singsong tone of voice and run
away. He described a childhood disrupted by recurrent episodes of illness. This meant
that his attendance at school was patchy, and he was behind in his development.
Although intelligent, he was slow to learn to read and write, a difficulty compounded
by what was later recognized as mild dyslexia. His schoolmates called him "thicko,"
and this sense of intellectual weakness stuck. Frequent absences also made it difficult
for him to form solid friendships in his early years. Later he made up the ground, academically and socially. By midadolescence he had a good network of friends at home
and had had a couple of successful relationships with girls. He did well in his exams
and was accepted by a university that he was excited to attend.

Bottom Line

Things had improved for Leo, but in spite of his successes he had not updated his bottom line, that is, his beliefs about himself remained fundamentally unchanged. His early experiences had left him with a fundamental sense of weakness and inadequacy—in his own words, "I am incapable." "Incapable" included a sense of physical fragility (the result of his early childhood illnesses), and also a feeling that he lacked the necessary qualities to be attractive to others. As his history might suggest, he saw himself as stupid, immature, and boring.

Rules for Living

Leo had developed a range of strategies designed to compensate for his perceived incapacity. He was a perfectionist in his work ("If I don't perform, people will think I'm stupid and laugh at me"). He worked equally hard at social relationships ("I must be interesting, or people won't want to know me"). He felt it necessary to keep a very careful eye on his health ("Unless I am vigilant, I could miss something serious"). And, especially when anxious or stressed, he kept a tight rein on every aspect of life that was possible ("Unless I'm in control, it could all fall apart")—an example of the rigidity under pressure that we referred to in our introduction and in Chapter 3 (p. 53). Despite his current difficulties, it was clear that to a substantial degree Leo's rules for living had been helpful to him—for example, his high standards had produced good quality work, and he could be a charming and entertaining companion.

Trigger Situations

Moving to consider Leo's difficulties from the perspective of low self-esteem elucidated how, at their heart, was a profound sense of himself as incapable, and a corresponding sense of vulnerability to harm. Leo's self-esteem could be seen as fragile rather than unvarying negative (i.e., he fell toward the middle of the continuum, described on p. 158). So long as he remained in a stable, familiar environment, all was more or less well. But the move to the university had created genuine demands and challenges (academic and social) that activated his underlying doubts about himself; strained his resources; made everything an effort; led to increasing stress, tension, and fatigue; and eventually created a feeling that his life was teetering on the verge of chaos. Furthermore, his failure to cope with ease seemed to him to confirm his negative sense of himself.

Maintenance Processes

Working on social phobia had tuned Leo in to the operation of anxious predictions, physiological signs of fear, and the role of avoidance and safety-seeking behaviors. Records he kept between sessions provided numerous examples of these processes in action. For example, when invited to meet fellow students in the college bar, he immediately assumed that they would find him boring and did not go (avoidance). He then took the fact that he had avoided socializing as further proof of how boring he was, rather than a natural consequence of his negative predictions (interpreting understandable inhibition in performance as evidence in favor of the bottom line). On another occasion he was required to hand in a piece of coursework. He predicted that it would not be up to the required standard and, after staying up most of the night to perfect it, spent much of his meeting with his tutor explaining at length that he had not been well and this was not a true reflection of what he was capable of (safety-seeking behaviors). The tutor then told him that in fact what he had done was just fine. Leo concluded that she must feel sorry for him and was just trying to be nice (discounting positive outcome). All these incidents appeared to him to confirm the bottom line. He became increasingly self-critical, felt worse and worse about himself, and was close to deciding that he might as well leave the university and go home; someone like him would never be able to make friends and be happy. It was at this point that he began to have thoughts of suicide.

APPLYING THE MODEL

To give you an opportunity to explore how this model might be useful in practice in approaching complex cases, and in particular comorbid anxiety and depression, we have included a blank version of the flowchart, with space to write, in Figure 8.4. If you are intrigued to discover how this framework might help to make sense of anxiety in relation to low self-esteem, then we suggest the following exercise:

1. Call to mind a specific patient who is anxious with whom you are working at the moment, *whom you would judge to have low self-esteem.* If possible, select a person you have quite a lot of information about, but whose story you have not yet formulated to your satisfaction. This is most likely to make the exercise clinically meaningful to you.

2. The blank flowchart provides an opportunity to formulate your patient's experience within the framework of the model of low self-esteem. What specifically fits under each heading? Be as accurate as possible, using what your patient has told you, and what you have observed in sessions. Aim to capture the idiosyncratic detail of your patient's experience at each stage of the development of current problems and how they are maintained.

3. Review your flowchart, using the following prompts to reflection if you wish:

- Does the developmental sequence make sense, with one thing following logically from another? As a simple rule of thumb, if you had had those experiences, within that context, would you have been likely to develop a similar bottom line, similar ideas about other people and your world, similar guiding rules for living? If not, where does the logic of the sequence break down? What do you think might be inaccurate or missing?
- At the maintenance level, are the elements in the vicious circle and the links between them clear? Can you identify your patient's anxious predictions word for word, or in clear images? How exactly do they experience anxiety (symptoms)? What maladaptive behaviors do they employ in different situations? Do you know how they experience confirmation of the bottom line? Words? An image? A wordless felt sense? A shift in emotional state? A gut feeling? Don't forget to look for environmental factors that might feed into the sense that the bottom line has been confirmed (e.g., criticism from others, or a partner unwit-

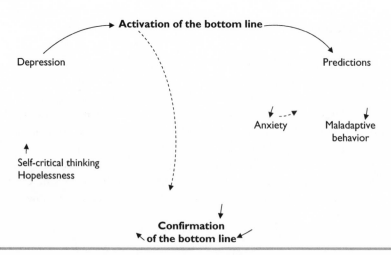

(Early) Experience *(x "wired in" factors)*
↓

The bottom line *(schema, basic or core belief)*
↓

Rules for living *(dysfunctional assumptions)*
↓

Trigger situations *(critical incidents)*
Situations in which the rules:
Are broken (no doubt) ↙   ↘ *Might be* broken (uncertain)

Activation of the bottom line

Depression   Predictions

                                        Anxiety   Maladaptive
                                                     behavior

Self-critical thinking
Hopelessness

**Confirmation
of the bottom line**

FIGURE 8.4. A cognitive model of low self-esteem: Worksheet.

tingly contributing to a sense of uselessness by trying too hard to help). And what about self-criticism and hopelessness? Can you specify these thoughts? And describe in detail how this person experiences depression?

- Are there gaps? Discrepancies? Things that do not fit? As we said in Chapter 3, a case formulation is always a draft: We can never know everything or reduce a person's life to a simple flowchart. Mark gaps, discrepancies, and so on with question marks—how could you explore them further?

- Does the flowchart make sense of the patient's presenting problems? Can you see how the patient might have come to have these particular difficulties, given the pattern that emerges?
- And does it make sense of difficulties that have arisen in therapy? Problems with engagement, perhaps, with homework completion, with the approach of termination, or with maintaining gains? Or perhaps difficulties in the therapeutic relationship—the patient's difficulties, or yours, or both?

4. When you have completed the flowchart according to the best of your knowledge at present, stand back a little and reflect on what you have done. How did this differ from how you might normally have formulated this case? What was included or excluded that normally would not be? What was helpful about the exercise? What did you learn, about the patient, and also about the process of formulating anxiety disorders within a low self-esteem framework? And what in your view were the shortcomings of the approach, in this particular case? Finally, consider whether there is anything from this that you could incorporate into your clinical practice, and if so, make a note of whom you will use it with, and when.

INTERVENTIONS DESIGNED TO ENHANCE SELF-ESTEEM

Low self-esteem, like other beliefs, is supported by biases in perception and interpretation that encourage the persistence of the system. People with low self-esteem are likely to be exquisitely sensitive to anything that is consistent with their negative self-view (e.g., errors, failures, signs of disapproval), while finding it hard even to notice information that contradicts it (e.g., successes, signs that others find them attractive). The information that penetrates this filter is also subject to bias (e.g., discounting, distorting, or making an exception of information inconsistent with the prevailing view; blaming oneself when things go wrong while attributing positive events to external factors; overgeneralizing from the negative). The literature on schema maintenance (e.g., Padesky, 1994; Young et al., 2003) and on attributional style (e.g., Alloy et al., 2004) elaborates exactly the kind of cognitive processing biases at work in low self-esteem.

Treatment interventions useful in working with low self-esteem are designed in essence to address these processing biases. Some broaden the view by directing attention toward information inconsistent with the old perspective (and consistent with new, more kindly and accepting ideas), whereas others work to question the negative meanings automatically attached to experiences. The model offers an opportunity to understand the system and points toward key targets that therapy will need to address. So it suggests that people like Leo who follow the anxious route to the righthand side of the maintenance vicious circle (Figure 8.2) will need to question and test anxious predictions, drop safety-seeking behaviors and reverse avoidance (see Chapter 6), as well as exploring alternative interpretations for events they would normally take to confirm of the bottom line. Working with this particular sequence is absolutely central to the treatment of anxiety. The model also suggests that questioning self-critical and hopeless thoughts may be necessary, and that (in some cases) we may need to start by treating clinical depression.

The fundamental principles of cognitive therapy outlined in classic texts (e.g., Beck, 1995), and ideas and methods drawn from established, evidence-based treatments for anxiety and depression prove invaluable here. They offer opportunities to break into maintenance processes at different points, using analysis of specific day-to-day experiences to open up options for responding less self-destructively to events that activate the bottom line. Thus they encourage hope that change is possible. Work at the maintenance level also begins the process of throwing unhelpful rules for living into sharp focus and fostering metacognitive awareness of the bottom line as a belief, a product of experience, rather than "the truth" or "me" (see Chapter 4). Particularly if we adopt the sandwich principle (Chapter 3, p. 64), ensuring that changes in particular thoughts and behaviors are explicitly linked to broader assumptions and beliefs, specific interventions can begin to chip away at and weaken the bottom line and the rules that support it, right from the outset. Once we begin to work on these in their own right, the wide repertoire of methods for changing and updating long-standing core ideas also become relevant (e.g., formulating and testing new assumptions, continuum work, historical test, reframing early memories, etc.).

It is not our intention further to elaborate established cognitive-behavioral methods here, with the exception of two sections below. One provides a systematic sequence of questions that can be used to undermine "evidence" supporting the bottom line; the other outlines new ideas for creating and strengthening new, more helpful, and accepting perspectives on the self. Readers who are interested in exploring the established methods in more detail are referred to texts such as Beck and colleagues (1979, 1985); J. S. Beck (1995); Hawton and colleagues (1989); Simos (2002); and Westbrook, Kennerley, and Kirk (2007). Patients can learn to use these tried and tested cognitive-behavioral techniques to change their own bottom lines by following self-help books such as Greenberger and Padesky (1995) and—specifically in relation to self-esteem—Fennell (1999, 2006b).

QUESTIONING THE BOTTOM LINE: UNDERMINING THE EVIDENCE

People who think badly of themselves do so for good reason. That is, a negative bottom line is not something we are born with—it is something we acquire through experience. Thus, as far as the person with low self-esteem is concerned, it is based on good evidence. The exact nature of the evidence varies from person to person, and once therapist and patient know what it is, they can begin to investigate the validity of the bottom line, and to formulate a more accepting and realistic alternative. Some common sources of evidence are summarized in Figure 8.5 on pages 170–171. The figure also shows how the kind of evidence people think supports their bottom lines is closely linked to unhelpful rules for living (examples will be found in the righthand column).

Once the main sources of evidence are clear, therapist and patient can begin to deconstruct the line of reasoning leading from experience to a global negative self-judgment using questions such as those illustrated in Figure 8.6. The text in italics describes an illustrative case example. The patient had developed severe, intractable PTSD following a relatively minor assault. It emerged that aspects of the circumstances under which the assault occurred "mapped on to" aspects of childhood experiences of sexual abuse (time of day, weather conditions, the physical makeup of the assailant involved in the assault). The patient had always suppressed the memory of the abuse; the accident opened Pandora's box, and he was unable to close it again. Identifying his powerful negative sense of himself and beginning to work on it gradually gave him the courage to begin to work on trauma memories, recent and long past.

The questions can provide a systematic framework for investigating how well the old view of self holds good, for formulating a possible alternative, for identifying how such an alternative might play out in everyday changes in thinking and behavior, and for preparing for the possibility of reactivation of the old system by future events. This last point is based on the assumption that old patterns are never entirely "deleted from the hard disk" but can be reactivated by appropriate constellations of stimuli. Action planning, using what has been learned in therapy, is potentially a useful preparation for this (see Chapter 10) and may also reduce anxiety about relapse. We should add that of course the sequence does not incorporate all the possibilities for undermining old belief systems—how therapists go about this task is bounded only by their own theoretical and clinical knowledge and their creativity, and by the characteristics and history of the individual patient.

Readers may wish to explore the utility of the sequence by bringing to mind a particular patient who is anxious and has low self-esteem with whom they would like to begin this work, and working through the questions in relation to that person. Because of its close alliance with depression, low self-esteem can have a certain "adhesiveness" that sometimes contaminates the therapist's thinking and makes it hard to see clearly how things might change. Following the questions through, perhaps with the help of a colleague who has some distance from the client, can help to open up new avenues. Ultimately, of course, it is the patient who needs to find new perspectives and ways forward, but freeing up one's own thinking as a therapist can be a helpful step along this route.

CREATING A NEW BOTTOM LINE

Like the ideas summarized in the previous section, many of the methods described in the cognitive therapy literature focus primarily on weakening and undermining old, unhelpful thoughts, assumptions, and beliefs. As we said earlier, this work will be more or less difficult, depending on how long-standing, entrenched, and generalized old patterns are, and on whether the patient has access to functional alternatives to the bottom line.

New developments, rather than focusing on undermining the old system, highlight the importance of establishing and strengthening new, more positive perspectives, especially with people whose problems are recurrent and of long standing. Clinical experience suggests that, for some of these people, working to deconstruct the old system can lead to an intensification of depressed mood, and even suicidality, which stand in the way of constructive change. Moving to construct a new alternative (as is done in the second half of the question sequence above) can provide a way out of this impasse. The work of Christine Padesky (Mooney & Padesky, 2000), Paul Gilbert (2005a), and Deborah Lee (2005) have been particularly influential here. Mooney and Padesky suggested awakening client creativity by accessing not simply new ideas (a new bottom

"Evidence" category	Further detail	Related rules for living (examples)
The fact of being ill (physical, emotional)	Anxiety itself can help to establish or reinforce the bottom line: "The very fact of being anxious means that there is something wrong with me *as a person*."	"I should always control my emotional state." "If I am anxious, then I'm pathetic."
Specific symptoms	In social phobia, for example, symptoms of anxiety are seen by the patient as extreme and glaringly obvious to others, even when in fact they may be imperceptible. They seem like a red flag signaling personal inadequacy to the observer.	"If I shake/blush/sweat/etc., then I am unacceptable." "I must do everything I can to conceal signs of anxiety" (→safety-seeking behaviors).
Failure to overcome difficulties	The case of late-onset PTSD outlined on page 158 is in part an example of this. One element of the picture is shame about not having successfully overcome the problem without help. Such feelings can prevent people from seeking therapy and make it difficult for them to engage even when they do so.	"I should always stand on my own two feet." "I should be in control of my feelings, not my feelings in control of me." "I should be able to deal with whatever comes my way."
Past errors and failures, bad acts (including the way life is now, given current strategies)	It is rare (if not impossible) to negotiate life without on occasion taking actions one later regrets, making mistakes, and messing things up on occasion. People with low self-esteem may see these human imperfections as further evidence of lack of worth, and fear of exposure can produce a persistent sense of insecurity. In particular, dysfunctional patterns that have genuine adverse consequences for how life is lived, sometimes extreme, may be seen as evidence of personal failure or badness, rather than an inevitable consequence of earlier learning, which the patient is now courageously trying to change.	"If I do something bad, that makes me a bad person." "If I make a mistake, then I am a failure." "If I have done something bad, then I should be punished." "If I have done something bad, then I deserve everything bad that happens to me."
Specific problems	The patient sees specific problems (such as anxiety disorders) as evidence of global inadequacy, rather than particular unfortunate patterns, learned through experience, which it might be possible to change. One woman, for example, who had genuine difficulties with self-assertion, viewed this as a sign of global inferiority rather than as an understandable reflection of her experiences early in life.	"If I have a problem, it means there is something wrong with me as a person."
Personal characteristics, physical or psychological	Physical characteristics include, for instance, shape and weight, skin color, disfigurement, and obvious physical disability. Failing to meet social norms of slimness (for women) or muscularity (for men) might, for example, induce a global sense of inferiority or freakishness. Failing to meet cultural norms can have a similar effect, for example, if one is strong and assertive as a woman in a setting where women are expected to be quiet, compliant, and submissive.	"If I am different, there must be something wrong with me. I should fit in."

Source	Description	"Evidence" statements
Comparison with others	Western European and American societies are highly competitive, not only in terms of performance but also in terms of material goods. It is rare to be at the top of every pile, and there are always people to whom we can compare ourselves unfavorably. With low self-esteem, coming second in a comparison is seen as a reflection of personal worth. Even those who have done well can worry constantly about a future fall.	"If someone is better at something than me, I am no good at all." "If someone is better off than me, I cannot be happy."
Others' problems	Taking excessive responsibility for the well-being of others may lead to anxious hypervigilance for signs that all is not well, overprotection, intrusiveness, and sharp self-blame if anything goes wrong for them. Parenthood and being an oldest sibling are particularly fertile soil for this line of reasoning.	"I am 100% responsible for the well-being of people I care for." "If someone has a problem, it's my fault and up to me to put it right." "If I fail to protect those close to me, then I am a failure as a parent/child/partner/friend/person."
Others' behavior towards self (past and/or present)	Past maltreatment, bullying, or abuse lays the ground for a pervasive negative sense of self, as well as for anxieties about failing to please or attracting further harm. Similarly, current bullying or abuse can lead to high levels of anxiety and undermine even a robust sense of self.	"If someone treats me badly, I must have done something to deserve it." "If someone criticizes me, that person is right."
Life circumstances or events (past and/or present)	Persistent adversity can provide a sense of being in some way doomed to struggle.	"Bad things always happen to me." "If I am not vigilant at all time, who knows what might happen?"
Cultural/religious values	For example, some groups within the Christian religion espouse a belief system that demands much while simultaneously castigating failure to measure up. Little allowance is made for love, forgiveness, compassion, or human frailty. People can be left with a persistent sense of failure and fear of punishment, not only in this life but the next.	"If I cannot do what is expected of me, that reflects my essential weakness and sinfulness."
Membership of a minority group that is a target for discrimination	If one belongs to a group that attracts criticism, rejection, and abuse from the surrounding larger society, it can be hard to maintain a sense of self-worth. Examples include racial, cultural, and religious minorities, the physically and mentally disabled, the disfigured, and the old.	"If I am treated badly, then that is a sign that there is something wrong with me."
Emotional reasoning	Statements like "It just feels true" reflect an assumption that powerful feelings have real truth value, rather than simply being powerful feelings. Such feelings are perhaps based on implicit memory traces resulting from highly emotional learning experiences early in life ("memory without awareness," see Chapter 5). Because the events on which they are based cannot voluntarily be called to mind, the resultant self-judgement "feels" vividly true, here and now.	"If something feels true, then it is."

FIGURE 8.5. Sources of "evidence" supporting the bottom line.

1. What is your client's bottom line? ("I am . . .")

   I am bad. I am worthless.

2. What sources of evidence does your client use to support the bottom line? There may be more than one. List them and then highlight the most influential.

   The fact that he was sexually abused between ages 8 and 12. Then, when he pushed away the abuser (a much older man), the latter fell, injured himself, and, 6 weeks later, died of a heart attack. The patient blamed himself for allowing the abuse to happen and felt responsible for the abuser's death.

3. Do you, the therapist, agree that the line of reasoning is valid, that is, that what the patient sees as evidence for the bottom line does indeed support it? If not, why not? What are the flaws in the argument? How else might the "evidence" be interpreted?

   No, I do not agree that this line of reasoning is valid. A child is not responsible for the abusive behavior of an adult, and he was terrified that the abuser would harm his family if he told them what was happening. He was not responsible for the abuser's death—there was probably no connection between the fall and the subsequent heart attack, and in any case his intention was not to harm, but simply to protect himself.

4. What disconfirming evidence, past and present, is your client ignoring, discounting, distorting, or seeing as an exception?

   He is ignoring his adult knowledge about the adult's responsibility for childhood sexual abuse—an issue now much in the news. He is also ignoring how young and frightened he was. He loved his family and wanted to protect them. If this was another person, not himself, he would not blame them. He is discounting aspects of himself that contradict his perception of himself as bad and worthless—for example, his successful career in a helping profession, his loving marriage, his contented children, his network of friends, his creative energy as a part-time artist.

5. Taking 3 and 4 into account (i.e., in the light of *all* the evidence available), what might make a more balanced (realistic, helpful) bottom line?

   The tentative alternative that the patient moved toward in therapy was, "I was a victim of abuse—it was not my fault. His death was probably nothing to do with what I did—and even if it was, I did not intend to harm him, even then. I am OK—he was bad."

6. What does the client need to do to bring the new perspective to bear in everyday life?

   - What information does he or she need to collect to counter the perceptual bias in favor of the old bottom line and strengthen the new, more positive perspective?

     Evidence of "OK-ness" (i.e., evidence in direct contradiction to his ideas of himself as bad and worthless). For example, feedback from clients in his workplace (he was an attentive and caring clinician), specific interactions with family and friends, positive reactions to his artwork, and his own satisfaction with it. The patient also began to collect evidence that being treated badly bore little or no relation to the worth of the person on the receiving end—for example, Christ, Nelson Mandela, innocent casualties of war.

   - What new rules for living might be more consistent with the new perspective, and more helpful?

     Just because something bad is done to you, it doesn't follow that you are either bad or worthless. It says more about the person who does it than it does about you.

   - What behavioral experiments would test the usefulness of the new rules, and validate the new bottom line? What safety-seeking behaviors does the client need to drop? What "risks" does he or she need to take?

     To be more open about himself in general, initially at a small level (he tended to conceal his true feelings for fear of rejection). To allow people closer, giving and receiving affection openly. To tell his wife and one very close friend about his experiences of abuse (he feared that they would agree with his judgment of himself as bad and worthless). To allow himself to think about the past instead of trying to shut it back in its box, and to experiment with feeling compassion for his child self rather than condemning him.

(continued)

FIGURE 8.6. Reevaluating the "evidence" for the bottom line.

These experiments were highly anxiety provoking, as the reader may imagine. Nonetheless, they provided an opportunity for the patient to realize that confronting the monsters did not leave him in fragments, and this led to a new and more hopeful rule: "Even when bad things happen, life goes on."

- What changes does the client need to make to behave *as if* he or she was worthy of respect and love (e.g., time for self, treats)?

   To reduce pressure on himself, rather than working all the hours God gave. To begin to express his own needs, likes, and dislikes and to meet them. To take time to relax and enjoy small pleasures. To be kind to himself, and to ask for comfort from others close to him when frightened and upset.

7. When the old system is reactivated, what does the client need to do to not get sucked back into it? What events might trigger the old bottom line? What cues might act as early warning signals that all was not well (e.g., changes in mood, particular trains of thought, patterns of interaction with others)? Draft an action plan.

   Triggers: Being overtired, reminders of the abuse (including external stimuli and his own feelings and sensations), stress.

   Cues: Tension, anxiety, becoming irritable, wanting to shut himself away.

   Action: Go back to therapy notes and identify things that can help to restabilize himself. Remember that the old bottom line is just an idea, developed for understandable reasons, not the truth. Keep working to strengthen the new perspective, until accepting himself as he is becomes second nature. Ask wife for help. Recontact therapist if necessary.

FIGURE 8.5. *(continued)*

line), but a vivid vision of how the client would like things to be, elaborated in multisensory, emotionally charged detail. This can then be consolidated and made real through specific changes in everyday thinking and behavior, with the vision providing a source of energy and motivation to move forward. Gilbert and Lee too use imagery, as well as enactive methods, to foster a sense of "safeness" that allows the work of tackling avoidance and safety behaviors to proceed, to repair deficits in clients' ability to soothe and comfort themselves, and to help them to reduce self-attack by developing "compassionate mind." These new approaches can be used to complement established methods more strongly aimed at deconstructing old perspectives and may, indeed, emerge as independent treatment approaches especially helpful to those we find most difficult to treat.

CONCLUSION

Understanding how low self-esteem develops and how it is maintained allows us to place specific anxieties within a broader transdiagnostic context that encourages a coherent approach to comorbidity, especially those cases where multiple anxieties may coexist with depression. The cognitive model of low self-esteem illustrates how anxiety and depression might be fed by (and feed) central negative beliefs about the self, and how the impact of treatment might be enhanced by understanding better the interrelationships between them, and working to ensure that changes in the one encourage simultaneous changes in the others.

NINE

Dealing with Uncertainty

In this chapter we consider another attitude that can consistently interfere with progress when people are anxious: the attitude toward the future. People who are anxious are highly likely to have experienced many intensely distressing events in the past, but so are other patients. This does not distinguish them from others who seek psychological help. However, their attitude to the future, and especially their inability to tolerate uncertainty, is a more consistent distinguishing feature. Sometimes this is relatively easily changed, for example, when someone carries out behavioral experiments that help them directly to resolve their uncertainties. When it is a more deep-seated attitude, and so resistant to change, intolerance of uncertainty contributes to the maintenance of current worries and fears and also to the development of new ones as situations and circumstances change.

MAKING SENSE OF ANXIETY AND UNCERTAINTY

In Chapter 3 we described three common reactions to anxiety: trying to keep control; rigidity of mind, body, and behavior; and safety-seeking activities. All three can also be understood as reactions to uncertainty. These reactions may have short-term benefits, such as making things feel more predictable, more under control and "safer," but they also contribute to the maintenance of anxiety. Theoretically, it follows that our treatments for anxiety will improve if we develop the skills needed to help people become more curious, more flexible, and more willing to explore despite their doubts and uncertainties.

Anxiety is about the threats, risks, or dangers that might or might not occur at some time in the future. One can never be sure that everything will be alright. Feeling anxious makes disasters seem more likely, and when disasters seem likely, anxiety increases (Butler & Mathews, 1983; Williams, Watts, MacLeod, & Mathews, 1997; Yiend, 2004). The link between thoughts and feelings operates in both directions. Even when something unpleasant is certain (you are about to have a tooth extracted, for example), elements of uncertainty remain, and a seemingly endless questioning process can be set in motion. How much will it hurt? How will you react? Will you be able to cope with the pain and the mess? Will you make a fool of yourself, or be able to get yourself home safely? If not, who could you call on? Would they be able or willing to help? This questioning process reflects both sides of anxiety: the perceived threats and the perceived ability to cope with them. When there is an imbalance between perceived threats and perceived resources, anxiety naturally follows (as described in Chapter 2), and attention is directed toward the business of making things feel under control, safe, and sure once again.

In general, the greater the uncertainty the greater the tendency to worry and the more likely that people will feel stressed by its cause (threats to a close relationship, to a job, or to financial security) as well as by the worrying itself ("I can't sleep for worrying"). People with GAD, which is defined in terms of worry, find it especially hard to tolerate uncertainty (Dugas, Gagnon, Ladouceur, & Freeston, 1998). Indeed, they probably occupy the other end of the continuum to sensation seekers and high-risk takers. But uncertainty is hard to tolerate for others as well, most obviously perhaps those who are plagued by obsessional doubts, or by the meaning of changes and sensations in their bodies (those with health anxiety). Uncertainty, as illustrated in the examples below, may also bring anxiety with it as part of a complex of apparently more serious or more pressing problems such as severe depression or self-harming behaviors. All of these versions of uncertainty can lead to the same reactions: attempts to keep things under control, rigidity, and avoidance.

Two points follow. First, certainty is not an option. Anxiety is about the future, and the future necessarily involves a degree of uncertainty. In therapy one of our aims is to help people face the (uncertain) future while suffering less from fear. Developing ways of helping them to accept and to tolerate their uncertainties may, therefore, help them to feel less anxious. Second, the number of potential worries is infinite. However good our techniques, those who find it hard to tolerate uncertainty will probably find something else to worry about when one worry is resolved. In treatment, therefore, we need to help people to attend to processes that maintain their fear of uncertainty, and to work at a metacognitive level (see Chapter 4). We should help people to reflect on their thinking processes: work with the underlying meaning of events (see Chapters 2 and 5), and with developing different attitudes to doubt and uncertainty.

A summary of the typical manifestations of uncertainty in different types of anxiety is provided in Figure 9.1. Our current hypothesis is that there are important similarities in the effects of uncertainty irrespective of diagnosis, and additionally there are many patients with atypical or mixed problems. For these reasons this chapter focuses on ways of helping people who find it hard to tolerate uncertainty irrespective of diagnosis. As yet there is insufficient research for us to know whether the same methods are valuable across some, or even all, diagnostic groups. However, when therapy becomes stuck, or when working with apparently treatment resistant cases, it is useful to have a broad range of methods available.

Given the huge range of sources of uncertainty it is not surprising that sometimes standard treatments for specific anxiety disorders are hard to apply and may not quickly produce expected results. Idiosyncratic susceptibility to uncertainty may not be as irrational as it appears, and careful case formulation work, the first step in any complex treatment, may help to derive hypotheses that make sense of it, often in terms of lessons learned in the past (see Chapter 3).

Generalized anxiety disorder: Anticipating and worrying about numerous negative possibilities: "What if . . . ?" Repeated catastrophization and poor decision making, as worry spreads from one topic to another. Attention is oriented toward worry about an uncertain future rather than toward problems and solution seeking.

Social phobia: Uncertainty is inherent in not knowing what other people might say or do, not knowing what they think of you, or wondering whether you have done or will do something embarrassing or humiliating.

OCD: Doubts about safety, about causing harm, or about failing to prevent harm predominate. Compensatory rituals, repetitive behaviors, rumination, and reassurance seeking can all be seen as attempts to make things more certain.

Health anxiety: Doubts about the meaning of changes in physical state, sensations, and internal cognitive or somatic phenomena. Catastrophizing about the possibility of having an illness or becoming ill. Never being sure that one is perfectly well.

Panic and agoraphobia: Not knowing whether or when your symptoms might suddenly escalate, or whether you will be able to cope with them, for example, when alone, or in an unfamiliar place. Uncertainty about whether others will help.

Simple phobias: Uncertainty about whether or when the feared object or situation might occur. Uncertainty about whether safety-seeking behaviors will be sufficiently successful, or about what might happen if attempts to protect oneself fail.

PTSD: The overgeneralized sense of danger makes bouts of intense anxiety unpredictable. Uncertainty about the meaning of symptoms, and recurrence of the traumatic event.

In general, anxious people interpret ambiguous information (uncertainty) linked with their individual sense of vulnerability in terms of threat, risk or danger.

FIGURE 9.1. Manifestations of uncertainty in different Axis I diagnoses.

Rob's uncertainties centered on a fear of anger. His father had an explosive temper, and as a small child Rob had been terrified about where the anger might be directed. He literally believed that "If he really lets it fly I could be snuffed out." He said his social life was dominated by "shoulds and musts," geared to limiting uncertainty about how others might react, and by trying to ensure that other people's reactions were predictable.

As the example shows, lessons learned in childhood contribute to shaping cognitive structures and cognitive/affective/behavioral patterns that persist into adulthood. Ways of making sense of these are described in more detail in Chapter 3.

ANTICIPATING AND AVOIDING COMMON PITFALLS

Patients who are anxious often put their therapists under pressure to provide reassurance. Many patients want to be sure—or to be reassured—that nothing too terrible will happen, if their symptoms continue to escalate, if they stop using safety-seeking behaviors, or venture into subjectively dangerous situations. Therapy inevitably introduces additional sources of uncertainty, so therapists should be clear about their own attitudes toward it and attempt to adopt an attitude of confidence while openly accepting the uncertainty. It is better for instance to say, "Yes, I can try to help you" than to say "Yes, I can help you." It is more truthful to say that "Most people gain much from therapy" than to imply that recovery is possible or likely (for details of results commonly obtained in ordinary clinical practice, see Westbrook & Kirk, 2005). It is important to remind people that doubts, uncertainties, and worries will always be there, and that therapy will focus on helping people to deal with them better, and not on attempting to remove them. The aim is to normalize the discomfort that uncertainty brings, not to suggest that it can always be faced with equanimity. Although cognitive-behavioral therapists are now well armed with theories, an evidence base for their methods, and good training, uncertainties about the success of their methods in individual cases remain.

The main point is that uncertainty is inevitable, and there is a danger in claiming that we know more than we do, or that there is a right way of proceeding that should invariably lead to a good outcome. Being aware of these uncertainties, and acknowledging them, fits well with the philosophy that informs the cognitive-behavioral approach. There are times when accepted protocols work well, and there are times when they do not. This needs explicitly to be recognized when faced with a patient's persistent anxiety despite one's own best efforts as a therapist. Reminders of the main strategies available to therapists working under conditions of uncertainty are summarized below.

- In general, work to foster curiosity, flexibility, and acceptance, rather than control, rigidity, and avoidance.
- Give people time: to think, rethink, respond to difficult questions, understand what is meant, build sufficient trust, disclose painful material, and so on.
- Do not claim to know more than we do. Not everyone can be helped by cognitive therapy.
- Double-check when in doubt: information, ways of understanding it, whether explanations have been understood, whether important material has been omitted.
- When in doubt about what someone means by what he or she says, ask for clarification. Listen occasionally to tapes of your therapy sessions.
- Remain curious: Make good use of the experimental method to gather data and evaluate it.
- Direct attention to material, topics, or areas that are otherwise ignored.
- Pay attention to the moment-to-moment process of therapy; watch for idiosyncratic signs of uncertainty and anxiety within the relationship and so on.
- Make an effort to understand different cultural attitudes, whether these stem from differences in ethnicity, place of origin, sex, age, and so on, so as to reduce confusion and uncertainty in communication, expectations, or assumptions.
- Remember that therapists too see things through their own theoretically, culturally, and individually determined frameworks.
- Acknowledge exceptions to the rule. For example, it is best for a patient to seek safety if violence in a relationship threatens to escalate. It is better to curb one's curiosity if it threatens to override recognition of risk when using street drugs or engaging in unsafe sexual practices.
- Use supervision (and colleagues) as sources of a second opinion, and also to assist in the process of developing skills of self-reflection.

Bearing these in mind provides appropriate setting conditions for helping patients to deal better with their own uncertainties.

Three sets of practical strategies are described next. First, we discuss those based on standard applications of cognitive therapy, which sometimes require modification when difficulties arise. Second, we focus on those derived from the treatment of worry and intolerance of uncertainty in generalized anxiety disorder. Third, we describe ways of helping people to live with uncertainty, drawn from a variety of sources.

STRATEGIES BASED ON STANDARD APPLICATIONS OF COGNITIVE THERAPY

Standard methods for working with dysfunctional assumptions and beliefs, including guided discovery and behavioral experiments, are often effective at changing fear of uncertainty at all levels of meaning. Occasionally, these methods do not work as expected, for example, if someone is persistently alarmed by the uncertainties of her experiences (such as having severe headaches, or a series of arguments with a partner). In these instances, it is important to unpack the meaning to her of the threat and its implications. Asking "What's the worst that could happen?" is a useful first step, as it helps the person to put her worst fears into words, and sometimes the worst fear is less terrible than the vague, unarticulated fear associated with the original uncertainty. The questioning can be pursued further by finding out more details about what someone is predicting, expecting, or supposing will happen. This can bring obvious exaggerations, guesses, or mind reading out into the open. However, there are two strategies that frequently do not help people in the process of reevaluating their negative predictions. The first is the attempt to define realistic probabilities for the specific threatening possibility. When a small amount of doubt (or uncertainty) is sufficient to maintain the anxiety, this has little effect, or only a temporary effect, and it is more useful to work with the meaning of the feared occurrence instead. This applies irrespective of whether the actual cost of the feared event is high (financial disaster, unemployment) or low (being late for a meeting, irritating someone) as the anxiety is linked to the perceived cost and determined by its subjective meaning.

The second strategy that is often frustrating is asking people for evidence for their predictions. The interactions between anxiety, negative predictions, and uncertainty about the future have been shown to bring into play a number of biases in information processing that together load the dice against other ways of thinking (e.g., MacLeod, 1996). The biases in question make it easy to think of the reasons why the feared outcome will happen and hard to think of reasons why not. They exacerbate the tendency to focus on negative outcomes rather than alternatives; they make it is easier to recall similar events, and to bring previous, anxiety-related judgments and impressions to mind. In addition, there is a proven two-way link between negative predictions and anxiety. Making negative predictions leads to increased anxiety, and feeling more anxious increases the tendency to make negative predictions. So looking for the evidence (for or against) is often less useful than using the prediction as a prompt to create appropriate behavioral experiments, and to evaluate their outcome in terms of relevant beliefs. As described in Chapter 3 (p. 64), it helps always to think in terms of the two slices of bread that help to hold the "sandwich" together: the beliefs and the behaviors, when working with complex cases.

A third standard method, Socratic questioning, may also be less useful especially when anxiety is linked to the experience of prolonged abuse during childhood.

Amy's childhood experiences involved unspeakable cruelty from which she escaped into a sequence of abusive relationships. When, at age 50, she decided to "take charge of her own life," her uncertainty about the conventions by which others lived caused her intense anxiety. This was especially the case with the ways in which people communicated with each other. Her uncertainties increased when she tried to break old patterns as she tended to veer from one extreme to the other: for example, she either revealed nothing about herself or much too much; she either said nothing to her new friends if they upset her, or castigated them so severely that she put good relationships at risk. Amy was unable to answer Socratic questions about how to behave within her current relationships. Questions such as, "What other options might you have?" "How else might you deal with this?" "How might someone else go about it?" were received with a blank expression (quickly followed by signs of despair). Given the childhood abuse, she had no store of functional material to draw on, especially concerning relationships. New information was acquired from her therapist and from others—through observation, reading, and inquiry; from literature, theater, and films, and through trying out different ways of behaving (experiment). Acquiring this new information was the product of behavioral work. Understanding its implications involved reflecting on Amy's beliefs, thus bringing both parts of the sandwich into play. Amy originally believed that it was dangerous to let anyone get close to her, or get to know her. As often occurs when starting to change a belief held with rigid conviction, at first she swung from one extreme to another. Learning to be flexible instead of rigid, and to modulate her behavior according to the situation, meant that she had to let go of another belief: that there was a single "right" way of doing things—that all she had to do to be able to engage better in social interactions was to learn the "rules of the game."

When Jane had her first child her uncertainties multiplied and interfered with her life profoundly. Her own mother had been neglectful and had failed to protect her from a physically abusive and alcoholic father. She had lived an isolated, impoverished, and frightened childhood and felt she had no idea how to behave as a mother—to the extent that she did not at first dare touch her baby for fear of causing harm.

Jane needed information about (good enough) mothering, about caring for infants and the many reasons for crying, and especially about changing diapers and cleaning the baby's genital area. These were not things she was able to work out for herself without help.

Such extreme cases clarify what is required before people can take advantage of standard cognitive methods. They also illustrate how the work that changes dysfunctional beliefs can be used at the same time to build, and to strengthen more functional ones. In less extreme cases, when people have had somewhat better experience of relationships, they may be able to draw on this experience to answer questions such as, "What if this happened to someone else?" or "What advice would you give another person you cared about?" Doing so could more readily help in the reevaluation of beliefs, for example, about being punished or ridiculed for "getting it wrong."

ACKNOWLEDGING THAT CHANGE INVOLVES TAKING RISKS

Jessie's parents apparently believed that praising children would spoil them and that constant correction and criticism would ensure that they became good and upright citizens. She learned to live as she thought they expected her to and later explained that she had never dared to "be herself." As an adult she was plagued by two sources of uncertainty. She said, "I don't know what it would be like to be me" and "I don't know how others would react if I didn't try to be the way they want." Her anxiety escalated whenever she tried to follow her inclinations, and whenever she forgot to maintain her hypervigilance for others' reactions. She struggled to build up an independent life and frequently sought reassurance from others, including her parents. Jessie had little sense of her own identity. Joint case formulation work revealed Jessie's view that she needed to please people to protect herself, but she did not at first understand how this linked with feeling worthless.

The strategic patterns of people like Jessie can often be observed in operation during therapy, but specific links with feelings are sometimes harder to specify, even though they may intuitively make sense. In Jessie's case the feelings of worthlessness were a product of "never being herself," so never feeling that she was appreciated for herself, but only for attempting to please people. She despised herself for doing this and concluded she had no personality. The difficulty for Jessie in changing this pattern was that she constantly had to balance current sources of anxiety (the fear of criticism, not knowing what others might do or say, being uncertain about how to keep others happy, not knowing how else to behave) with a new source of anxiety: the risk involved in changing her ways.

In such cases it may seem inevitable that anxiety increases before it diminishes, and it can be difficult to judge how much change someone is ready for or capable of at a particular time. Explicit discussion can resolve this issue, and reasons for making changes need to be clear before starting. It helps, for instance, to clarify the disadvantages of continuing in the present way, and to look at them together with the (as yet hypothetical) advantages of making changes. For someone like Jessie, who had little sense of her own identity, a period of exploration and experimentation is necessary, but during this time it is likely that such people will encounter further difficulties and make "mistakes" as they search for a new way to relate to people that works for them. They will be faced with ambiguity and doubt in ways that at first may make them feel more rather than less uncertain. It was when Jessie's pattern of pleasing people worked too well, and a colleague told her that he had fallen in love with her, that she felt ready to change. She was certain that she did not reciprocate his feelings—that she was tempted to listen to his words of appreciation, but also that doing so did not fit with her belief in being loyal to her current partner. The episode helped her to discover something about her own values and personality, and it contributed to taking the risks involved in changing her pattern of pleasing others.

Working with the Right Amount of Affect

When anxiety is too high it is difficult to focus attention on anything else. When too little anxiety is present (or when people avoid affect, as described in Chapter 7) there is too much detachment. But for change to come about cognition and affect need to be engaged. Presumably this applies during the therapy session, when talking about anxiety and also, subsequently, when the person who is anxious is attempting to apply what has been learned during the session. The window for change needs to be open, and people need to be able to look through it without being overwhelmed by their anxiety and unable to focus attention on anything else. If, for example, a homework assignment is carried out as planned but fails to make a difference, then therapists should ask for details about the focus of attention and level of affect at the time and should also consider observing the patient during the experimental work, either in the session or outside of it (see Chapter 6, pp. 109–110, for a discussion of the value of therapist-guided in-session behavioral experiments).

Foa and Kozak (1986) explained that for emotional processing to proceed and fears to be laid to rest, the whole cognitive-affective fear structure should be activated— almost as if this makes available all the necessary ingredients and processes for change. The implication is that unprocessed fears will remain "unfinished business" and continue to introduce doubts, uncertainties, and anxiety in the future. This does not, however, suggest that it is helpful to encourage patients to experience their anxiety at maximum intensity (so what does it mean then?)

STRATEGIES DERIVED FROM THE TREATMENT OF GAD

Much of what follows is based on methods developed for helping patients with GAD to deal with their worrying. According to Dugas and colleagues (1998), GAD has high intolerance of uncertainty as one of its main features. One of Dugas and colleagues' main aims was to increase flexibility and, as already mentioned, a large body of data demonstrates a close relationship between worry and rigidity. The hypothesis is that uncertainty makes people want to increase their sense of control, and attempting to achieve control reduces variability in their responses. Reduced responsiveness has been demonstrated in all the systems measured (cognitive, affective, behavioral and physiological; in recordings of the EEG, etc.). However, rigidity prevents adaptation, and the development of flexibility. Borkovec and colleagues (1993) also reminded us that worrying, and the rigidity that goes with it, precludes emotional processing and leaves people susceptible to alarming imagery. It is as if they switch on the cognitive system (the worrying) in preference to being bombarded with intrusive, and intensely evocative, memories and images. Although the worry feels bad, it feels less bad than being faced with raw, unprocessed, frightening images. So worry operates at least partly as a kind of avoidance. This description may not fit well with the subjective experience of low-grade worrying about completing daily tasks, for example, but the evidence is that it fits well for those with GAD. People who suffer from GAD endlessly ask themselves, "What if . . . ?" and answer their queries with thoughts of possible, more-or-less catastrophic disasters.

Acknowledging the Advantages of Worry

Worry, like uncertainty, has advantages as well as disadvantages, summarized informally as those of "alarm, prompt, and preparation" (see, e.g., Davey & Tallis, 1994; Wells, 1997, 2000). Worrying serves as an alarm system in that it alerts people to the possibility that something might be going wrong, it prompts them to take action, and it leads to anticipatory coping that serves as a preparation for dealing with difficulties when and if they arise. Many people have a "sneaking suspicion" that their worrying is useful that may contribute to explaining their superstitious statements, and possibly some of the ritualistic behavior, that often accompanies worry. Of course worrying also has disadvantages: It feels bad, spreads from one thing to another, becomes hard to interrupt, and makes it harder (not easier) to make decisions. It can irritate others, who learn to ignore it or find themselves repeatedly giving reassurance. It triggers thoughts about the possible harmful effects of the worrying, and of not being able to control it, or metaworry (Wells, 1997, 2002). It follows that attempts to tackle worry (or the uncertainties that underpin worry) should be firmly based on a recognition of its valuable aspects. Otherwise the patient and therapist will find themselves at cross purposes, homework assignments will not be completed, and commitment to therapy is likely to be half-hearted.

> Esther was in her 20s when her father died suddenly of an aneurysm. Since then she had become superstitious. Like many worriers, she said, "Unless I worry something is bound to go wrong." She also believed that thinking about things could make them worse—or even make bad things happen. When her grandson went traveling around the world she put a photograph of him in every room and thought good thoughts about him before she fell asleep at night. Her daughter was later than expected when paying her a visit, and Esther refused to eat a chocolate until she arrived "or something bad might happen to her." Each of these behaviors was intended to reduce her sense of being vulnerable to uncertainty and gave her a temporary (false) sense of control. Although she readily acknowledged that this control was illusory, she felt better trying to create the illusion, in a wide variety of ways rather than through excessive, obsessional repetition, than feeling constantly at the mercy of chance happenings. A two-part treatment strategy was useful: first, to help Esther to feel more in control where that was appropriate (her worrying had interfered with her ability to organize herself and to run her life), and second, when there was nothing to be done, to help her use calming and distracting methods, and to be more accepting of the uncertainty.

Dealing with the Process, not the Content

Worry spreads from one thing to another—especially in the middle of the night or at other times when there is little else to grab one's attention. Therapists often find that their efforts to deal with a patient's worries one at a time are eventually thwarted by the ways in which one worry is replaced with another. It is as if the beliefs and attitudes associated with the inability to tolerate uncertainty remain totally untouched. It can be useful to work through and to resolve one or two worries, but it is far more useful to help people to turn their attention toward dealing with the process of worrying rather than its content. A similar argument can be applied to dealing with the processes of reassurance seeking and rumination.

A basic, and simply described method for working on the process not the content is attention training (Wells, 2000). This involves practicing consciously switching attention between different sources of information (auditory, kinaesthetic, visual, etc.). Patients first learn to switch their attention during therapy and then practice doing this on their own, for about 10 minutes at a time, frequently and regularly. The aims of this method, and the precise techniques involved, are described in detail by Wells (2000, pp. 139–147). Preliminary findings from studies using it suggest that it is quick and effective, although the mechanism by which it works is not yet clear. However, it is important to consider the role of attention more thoroughly than is traditional in the standard treatments for specific anxiety disorders, particularly when working with more complex cases. At the very least, each of the techniques suggested below has the minimum effect of switching attention, and when attention changes, opportunities for new learning may also arise.

More overtly cognitive methods involve using guided discovery to help people to become more aware of the effects of worrying, and of being unable to tolerate uncertainty. Some questions for helping with this process are listed below, followed by some more ideas about how to help people interrupt and deal with the process of worry once it has started.

- "Have you always been a worrier?"
- "If we got that worry fixed, what would be the next thing?"
- "Could it be the worrying that's the problem rather than the thing you are worrying about?"
- "Is worry useful to you? In what way? How do you know?"
- "Are there times when you don't worry? What is different about them?"
- "What happens when you don't have a worry? How does that feel?"

Specific awareness training is sometimes also needed to help people to catch the worrying in its early phases. For example, it might help to use cues (such as mealtimes, an alarm clock set to ring at hourly or random intervals, telephone calls) to prompt people to tune in to their current level of worrying and to ask themselves such things as when this began, what triggered it, what disasters are they predicting, or what specifically is the worry about. The idea is that as soon as worrying comes to attention it should be interrupted. Otherwise it will continue with increasingly distressing and disruptive effects. Interrupting the process early is most likely to succeed and provide patients with an opportunity to find out more about the effects on them of the worry process. Worries (and, e.g., uncertainties about relationships) are often triggered by the content of therapy sessions, requiring sharp powers of observation in the therapist for signs that the patient is slipping into self-protective mode. Overt worry is obviously more readily noticed, but covert worry or uncertainty may continue for some time before it becomes clear that attention is divided. Once the rationale for interrupting

worry has been understood the process can be interrupted more easily without interfering with collaboration, and the interruption should be followed by an invitation to
reflect on the process there and then. First, it is useful to make sense of what happened:
to use case formulation work to relate the onset of worry to the idiosyncratic sense of
vulnerability that provokes anxiety in this person. Then the relevant risks, threats, and
safety-seeking behaviors can be identified more clearly, and appropriate plans for facing fears and reexamining thoughts about them can be made.

PRACTICAL TIPS

Three "tips" are described next for helping chronic worriers to stop worrying without
dealing with the content of their particular worry. The first of these is to pay attention
to the feelings experienced when worry is forcibly interrupted and to acknowledge
their variety. These range widely, for example, from frustration and irritability to relief.
Worry grabs attention, feels important, spreads from one thing to another, and makes it
hard to focus on anything else. As Wells (2000) reminded us, positive and negative
beliefs about worrying are relevant. Worriers often think that if they continue worrying
they will in the end arrive at a solution to their problems, and indeed occasionally solutions do occur during a bout of worrying. However, this seems to be mostly a chance
occurrence—and of course one that is highly reinforcing. It makes the habit of worrying
even harder to break. It is far more likely that worrying, when it is habitual, will activate a tendency to catastrophize and will fill the uncertain future with apparently realistic disasters. It increases cognitive rigidity when it is flexibility that is needed for finding new options and/or solutions. It includes an element of avoidance that if not faced
will maintain anxiety.

The second tip is to tackle positive beliefs about worrying. One simple and effective way to do this is to reflect on worrying that is obviously not useful, such as night-
time worry. At 3:00 A.M. worrying spreads easily from one thing to another, and the distress associated with it can escalate rapidly. Recognizing that this is not helpful can
help to throw doubt on the value of the process and help people to feel less compelled
to let it run on unchecked.

The third tip is to explore the possibility that the particular worry relates to some
"unfinished business" in the past. In some of the case examples we described so far,
such as those of Jessie and Amy, their current anxiety related to earlier experiences,
either during childhood or subsequently. Understanding the meaning to them of these
experiences can provide more information for the formulation, with more specific
implications for treatment (see Chapter 5).

Distinguishing Soluble from Insoluble Problems

Dugas and colleagues (2003) advanced our thinking about uncertainty and the various
ways of dealing with it by distinguishing between two sources of uncertainty. The first
arises out of worries about current problems such as interpersonal conflicts or financial
difficulties, and the second arises out of worry about hypothetical situations. For example, worrying about how to get through the next few weeks, days, or hours is different
from worrying that one day someone close to me will become seriously ill. To help with

current difficult times people can adopt more or less helpful strategies with a fair chance of success, at least intermittently. There is nothing they can do to change the probabilities of an illness striking someone they love. The methods of Dugas and colleagues for helping people deal with the uncertainty of future events in the first case are to train them in the use of problem-solving techniques, including problem orientation. For dealing with hypothetical worries, the methods they suggest are exposure to thoughts and images of the imagined threat. This may lead to habituation, or to other spontaneous cognitive change, as suggested in Chapter 5. Learning to accept the uncertainty and using mindfulness meditation is also likely to be helpful (see p. 188).

A simple method described by Butler and Hope (2007) can be used to start the process of deciding which type of uncertainty is involved. Figure 9.2 represents the worry tree. This is a decision tree that guides the worrier through three sets of questions. The ultimate purpose of this method is to help the person decide either to take appropriate action or to accept that there is nothing else he can do and let go of the worrying. Having first specified a particular worry (which admittedly is not always a simple matter), the person is asked to consider what action he could take, and then he is encouraged to make specific behavioral plans, using the steps illustrated in the figure. The value of this method is that it helps to initiate further action and to decide when there is nothing more to be done, and therefore that it is safe to let the worry drop.

There is evidence that worriers are slow to initiate the process of problem solving, or poor at problem orientation (e.g., Dugas, Letarte, Rheaume, Freeston, & Ladouceur, 1995). It is as if the worry intervenes and prevents them focusing properly on specifics—as indeed might be expected if it is operating as a kind of avoidance. Using the decision tree is one way of helping them to overcome this avoidance, and then they may not need any further problem-solving training. Research on people with GAD shows that their problem-solving skills are as good as those of others, but when caught up in worrying they do not start to use them. An example is provided by Lester, who suffered from GAD.

Lester was the oldest of three children and an affectionate and sensible child. When he was 12 his father left home, and his mother, who was stressed and depressed, had to work long hours to support the family. Lester took his sisters to school, walked them home each afternoon, made the tea, and tried to do everything possible to help his mother. He thought constantly ahead so as to make life easier for her, and in case something went wrong. For example, he worried that his sisters would dash across the road without waiting for him, or get into a fight, or get ill. His habit was to anticipate possible disasters. His motto, if he had had one, would have been "forewarned is forearmed." Lester had good problem-solving skills, but in adulthood he had also lost confidence in his ability to solve problems. Use of the worry tree played an important part in reviving his problem-solving confidence—with good reason. His experience had provided him with great problem-solving skill, but also with the sense that he could at any time be overwhelmed by something that it was beyond his powers to handle. Further work on his beliefs (his sense of vulnerability) using standard cognitive methods was also needed and helped him to recognize that sometimes he could solve problems effectively, but that some problems are not amenable to practical problem-solving methods.

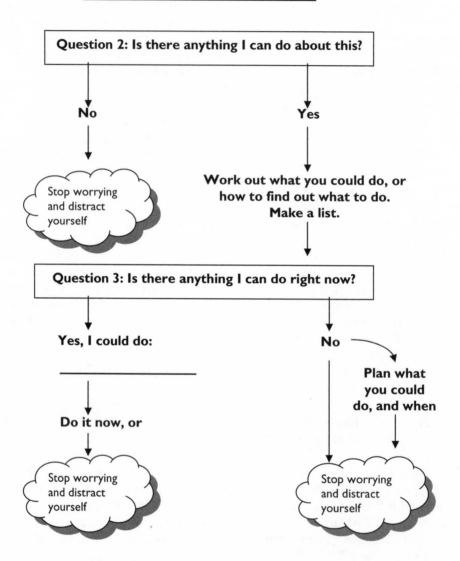

Now you know it is safe to let your worries drop.

FIGURE 9.2. The worry tree (Butler & Hope, 2007).

STRATEGIES FOR HELPING PEOPLE
TO LIVE WITH UNCERTAINTY

Most people need further help when it comes to dealing with hypothetical worries, and this is where general attitudes and assumptions concerning acceptance and normalization play an important role. Uncertainty has positive and constructive effects. There is nothing so deadening as routine, or being stuck in a rut—at least when you are not living with fear. Then novelty becomes interesting and the unexpected is enlivening, even when it involves risk. It also opens the mind to new possibilities—hence the argument that creativity is a fundamental survival skill and a source of solutions to problems (Simonton, 2005; Sternberg, 1998). Creativity and exploration are inhibited by too much novelty or by fear, stress, and anxiety. They are more likely to flourish under conditions of sufficient safety and freedom, such as those we strive to provide within therapy. This has been demonstrated in a series of experiments by Friedman and Forster (2001) using a task in which participants help a computer-simulated mouse trapped in a maze to find its way out. In one condition a piece of cheese is shown outside the maze; in the other an owl hovers above the maze. Participants shown the cheese maze subsequently solved more problems and generated more creative ideas than those shown the owl maze, and they also adopted a more adventurous processing style. Similarly, children—and supposedly adults also—are demonstrably more creative when their opinions are sought, their ideas respected, and they are encouraged to use their curiosity to play, to experiment, and to explore. People are more creative when in a good mood (for a summary of relevant findings, see Wade & Tavris, 1993). So uncertainty, curiosity, and creativity, under the right conditions, reduce the rigidity of fearful attitudes and lead to productive exploration. As Mooney and Padesky (2000) put it: "Ambiguity and doubt are critical ingredients in creative change."

Hypothetical worries can never be "solved," or resolved, in the way that problems are solved. Instead, we need to think about how to live with uncertainties. When therapists become too busy as problem solvers, it may give the wrong impression to people who are finding it difficult to live with their more deep-seated or existential uncertainties.

Clarifying What the Worry Is About

It is easier to live with specific difficulties than with vague, unspecified worries; the process of specification reduces some of the uncertainty. The imagination seems to expand to fill the gap when uncertainty remains high. People often use the language of "feeling worried" rather than the more cognitive language that is involved when they name the things they are worried about, or describe the cognitive processes of worry. Of course it is possible to feel worried, but the feeling does not arise out of nowhere. There is usually a reason behind it, and specifying the reason can start the process of removing one source of uncertainty. When vague worries persist, the instruction "out of the head and onto the paper" can be helpful. The following strategy can be applied to specific and to hypothetical worries. The aim is to write down what the worry is about. If the worry occurs at a time when it cannot immediately be attended to, or at night when trying to sleep, then writing it down puts the worry (quite literally) aside, for further consideration later. Imaginal methods of setting worries aside can also be helpful: putting them in a box and closing the lid; writing them on scraps of paper and letting them float downstream; putting them one by one on the bonfire and watching them go up in smoke; or just closing the book on them.

Borkovec's method of stimulus control (Borkovec & Whisman, 1996) is a more structured and sophisticated version of these ideas. He suggested setting aside a worry time, or a place to worry, or even a worry-free zone, and then when worries occur at other times, or if they occur in the worry-free zone, they are put aside. Gradually, and with repeated practice, the worry-free place or time can be expanded. Sometimes people discover that they are unable to find anything to worry about when the worry time arrives; or they can more successfully turn the worries into problems to solve, having deliberately brought them to mind. Of course it is also important to consider the meaning to people of not worrying, and helpful overtly to test the validity of the negative predictions that come to mind when worrying. Borkovec suggested keeping a diary in which negative predictions are specified and later linked to actual outcomes. The usual finding is that negative predictions made when worrying are exaggerated or false, and that the bad things that do happen have not usually been predicted.

Strengthening Incompatible Behaviors

The essence of the behavior incompatible with worry (and anxiety) described by Borkovec (2004) is to focus on the present moment: to attend without avoidance or reluctance to what is happening right now, accepting the present just as it is, and accepting all reactions and feelings in the present, just as they are (as in mindfulness-based cognitive therapy; Segal et al., 2002). Thinking about the future will bring uncertainty with it, and the nature of that future will be colored by the perception and anticipation of risks or threats. Accepted wisdom says it for us: "My life has been full of terrible misfortunes, most of which never happened" (a sentiment attributed both to Montaigne and to Mark Twain).

Anticipating misfortunes elicits painful reactions even though they have not occurred, and may never occur. Living in anticipation of disasters brings rigidity with it: It narrows the range of responses to the present. For example, Borkovec (2004) reported that cardiovascular reactions are reduced in people who suffer from GAD when the stimuli that provoke them are positive and when they are negative. As already mentioned, with intolerance of uncertainty comes a habitual reduced responsiveness that could theoretically be reversed by introducing a source of flexibility. Sources of more flexible responding have been sought traditionally in progressive muscular relaxation, and more recently in helping people to move toward adopting a more relaxed lifestyle. Other sources include mindfulness meditation, play, artistic expression, physical exercise, breathing exercises, and the kinds of interactions with others that can be achieved without keeping an eye out for problems and that therefore facilitate a sense of immediate personal contact.

Validation

In the context of developing ways of living with uncertainty, and for people like Jessie (see p. 180) who are uncertain about their identity, validation can play an important role. The methods have been well described, for example, by Linehan (1993a, 1993b),

Leahy (2001, 2003), and others. But validation is a more sophisticated tool than it at first appears. Pinel and Constantino (2003) described what is involved, and they drew our attention to two separate needs than can be met through the process of validation. The first is a need for positivity. People like to see themselves in a positive light, and indeed they prefer positivity to the truth about themselves. This seems to be the aspect of validation that many therapists understand most easily, and many of them develop ways of feeding back to their patients the positive, and functional things that they have observed about them. However, the other need is for verification: People like to feel that they are recognized for what they are, and to feel that they know themselves. Feedback that does not fit their experience of themselves is therefore discounted, and especially for people who have a poor opinion or a downright negative view of themselves, it can feel threatening to be presented with a positive view. For example, telling Jessie, whose childhood was filled with constant correction and criticism, about the positive qualities observed in her (such as humor, energy, willingness to cooperate, courage in facing difficulties), or asking her to list her positive qualities (with or without the help of others) was readily discounted. For validation to succeed, and for it to play a part in establishing the secure base that is needed for people to start to explore their worlds, it should not challenge the sense of knowing the self. So we need to learn how to balance the positivity with the verification: how to understand and validate someone's experience of being worthless or bad, for instance, without suggesting that this is the way we also see them. For Jessie this meant placing her attempts to be "nice" in the context of the unhelpful pattern of trying to please people, and recognizing that this was, as she put it "dishonest." Acknowledging the dishonesty (and formulating the reasons for it in terms of "not being true to herself"), enabled Jessie to start making more assertive choices in relations with others, the results of which enabled her to come to more valid conclusions about herself and her willingness to cooperate, ability to be humorous, and so on.

Using the Therapy Relationship

Cognitive therapists have been slow to openly discuss the various parts played in therapy by the therapy relationship. There has been a (productive) emphasis on collaboration, on the use of mutual feedback, and of engaging the processes of guided discovery, but little discussion of how to adapt to the needs of particular patients. In addition, we should recognize that the way in which we relate to a patient with more complex, long-standing problems has a particular meaning for them. This has been put into words well by Bateman (2000), and his views can be used to remind us to think about how we come across to others and about the meaning to our patients of the ways in which we relate to them:

> Part of the benefit which personality disordered individuals derive from treatment comes through experience of being involved in a carefully considered, well-structured and coherent personal endeavour. What may be helpful [. . .] above all is the experience of being the subject of reliable, coherent and rational thinking [. . .] experiences such as these are not specific to any treatment modality [. . .] they have an impact because these people have been deprived of exactly such consideration and commitment during their early development and frequently throughout their later life. (p. 21)

So we need to think about the ways in which we show our consideration and commitment. As cognitive therapists we need to make explicit our attempts at providing a carefully considered, well-structured, and coherent personal endeavor. The careful (joint) consideration is especially important when making sense is otherwise difficult. We can also misconstrue the effects of our interactions, and a useful safeguard is provided by listening regularly to tapes of the sessions we provide, and reflecting on the process as well as the content.

If our treatment-resistant patients who are anxious are going to be able to face their doubts and uncertainties then we need to consider how, within our relationship with them, we can provide conditions that will make this more likely. We need to provide the framework of security and stability that enables people to start to explore, in the therapy room and outside it. We need to think about how we build trust when trust is lacking, and about other factors such as our sense of timing when it comes to pushing people on, and about the judicial use of humor and playfulness when trying out new ways of behaving (as described in Chapters 6 and 7), perhaps especially in relation to other people (see Panksepp, 2004, for an account of the neuropsychological and confidence-building effects of play). Our own attitudes to mistakes, failures, puzzles, and predicaments are readily discernible, especially by those people who have spent much of their lifetimes on the lookout for other people's reactions. Denying or masking our confusion will not help.

CONCLUSION

Attitudes toward the treatment of anxiety, and especially toward the treatment of anxiety in the context of the various kinds of comorbidity and complexity that we have described in this chapter, mark a profound change from attitudes to anxiety management a quarter of a century ago—and even more recently than that. In particular they allow us to build on the evidence base in ways that are theoretically consistent and that release our own flexibility and creativity without losing touch with lessons learned earlier.

When helping people to accept their uncertainties it is tempting to recommend that they seek a balance: that they avoid the extremes, as if the "right" amount of fear and the "right" amount of uncertainty will allow them to use their capacities for adaptation and creativity in the service of finding solutions to troubles and difficulties. This would suggest that ambiguity and doubt should be kept within moderate levels, so there is neither so little that people become bored, nor so much that they become fearful. But these are not the only relevant dimensions, and our patients provide us with many useful lessons about anxiety. They often demonstrate that it is possible to be scared, doubting, and uncertain and still to do something new, and we should think more about the foundations of such courage. We should increase the attention we give to our patients' strengths and resources, and to the positive, functional beliefs that allow them to accept and to face their fears even when they cannot be certain of the outcome of doing so. Clearly we need more research on the determinants of such strength.

What kind of reassurance can we offer those whose lives are limited by living with fear and anxiety? Perhaps it is possible to offer a limited kind of reassurance—or assurance—that anxiety is normal, and that its processes and effects are useful as they motivate us to pay attention to possible sources of danger. We can learn individually when to ignore our fears (e.g., when plagued by doubts that "I ran someone over this morning," or convinced again that "this headache means I have cancer"). We can learn when to test out reality in the ways described earlier, and when to do our best to accept and live in an unpredictable world without letting it interfere with our ability to live productive lives. As social animals, we need each other, and the benefits of acknowledging, sharing, and accepting the different manifestations of anxiety, and the different ways of living with uncertainty, have yet to be fully recognized. Qualities of practitioners and of the ways in which they interact with their patients may, for example, be crucial. We now know that habits of attending selectively can be established in one set of situations and later revealed in others (Mathews & MacLeod, 2002). It has always been puzzling that spending a few hours with someone can make any difference at all. If doing so affects what they attend to, and the way in which they attend (e.g., nonjudgmentally, without avoidance or self-protection), then maybe this is not so surprising after all.

PART V
ENDING TREATMENT PRODUCTIVELY

"I'm afraid that I won't be able to manage without you."
"What shall I do if it comes back again?"

Even when progress has been good, patients are often concerned as the end of treatment approaches that they may be unable to build on what they have learned, or to deal effectively with setbacks, once sessions have come to an end. Equally, new learning may remain fragile if it is not consolidated and used as a basis for thinking ahead.

In this last chapter, we suggest a framework for systematically consolidating patient's new understanding, discoveries, and skills and using this information as a foundation for effective action planning for the future.

TEN

Creating a Therapy "Blueprint"

We have attempted in this book to provide some new resources for therapists who find that their patients who are anxious do not always respond as expected. Throughout we have drawn on our understanding of theory, on our knowledge of research, and on our clinical experience, in normal clinical practice as well as in research trials, to provide practical suggestions based on those that our patients have found useful. This approach has allowed us to revisit and to develop our ideas about issues and themes that are central to any discussion of the treatment of anxiety disorders, and that have informed the structure of the book. These include the value of in-depth assessment of idiosyncratic meanings, whether expressed in words, images, or through describing a less easily defined "felt sense." We show how such careful assessment lays the foundations for case formulation work that helps patients to make sense of their experiences, even when the picture is complicated by long histories and high comorbidity. We emphasize the importance to engagement of fostering decentering from emotionally charged cognitions (metacognitive awareness), and the crucial role of experiential methods such as working with imagery and memory, and behavioral experiments, in ensuring whole-person change. Finally, we identify transdiagnostic issues that help us as therapists to work more effectively with comorbity (avoidance of affect, low self-esteem, and intolerance of uncertainty).

The methods we have suggested throughout are intended to enhance the effectiveness of treatment when standard methods have limited success. They are held together by three general principles, first made explicit in our introduction, and again in Chapter 3: to encourage curiosity rather than control, to increase flexibility (and reduce rigidity), and to help people to approach, accept, and explore when they feel anxious, rather than to seek protection through avoidance or safety-seeking behaviors. Our intention as therapists is that our patients should develop this stance over the course of therapy, and that they should carry it with them when sessions come to an end.

One of the underlying assumptions of cognitive therapy is that therapists will aim to make themselves redundant by transferring to patients the knowledge and skills that they need to function independently. This aspect of cognitive therapy is underscored by external constraints on therapeutic contact, such as limitations in resources and the constraints imposed by insurance companies and managed care. Such constraints push therapist and patient to work at maximum efficiency, sometimes to the detriment of quality of care. Thus, in modern mental health care, managing termination constructively is a perennial concern, most particularly perhaps with less straightforward cases such as those that have been our focus in this book. In such cases, failure to prepare for the end of therapy can mean that important new learning is lost, that setbacks are responded to with fear and despair rather than viewed as an opportunity to learn more, or that the approach of treatment termination activates old schemas such as fears of abandonment or of being unable to cope alone.

In our concluding chapter, we address this problem by considering issues relating to ending treatment. We offer a practical framework that allows therapists and patients to look back to what has been learned, and to look forward to how new learning can continue after therapy has come to an end.

THE PROCESSES INVOLVED IN ENDING TREATMENT

Cognitive therapy shares with other therapeutic approaches a concern with patients' responses to ending treatment, and it is always important to address these responses explicitly and directly. This is especially so if patients' problems are of long duration or accompanied by hopelessness, if complications have made the work difficult, if patients' confidence that they can manage alone is still shaky, or if progress has not gone according to plan. So therapists should elucidate thoughts and feelings about coming to the end of treatment and work with these using standard methods. These include acknowledging the validity of feelings of doubt, loss, anger, or anxiety; using the formulation to make sense of patients' responses to termination; using verbal, behavioral, and imaginal methods to reevaluate them; and working to foster confidence that the transition to independence can be made successfully. One of the prime tasks of treatment is to facilitate generalization. This means to consolidate and extend gains, and to prepare people to manage future difficulties and setbacks using what they have learned.

Preparation for Ending

At the start of therapy there are numerous tasks to be completed, especially when comorbidity complicates the presentation. First and foremost is the need to establish a trusting working relationship, and it is important at this stage to remember to check out patients' expectations for therapy. These are often unrealistic, even though at some level people realize that they cannot expect to live without fear, stress, and anxiety. Discussion of expectations provides an opportunity to clarify the plans and intentions of both parties, as it reveals that the end point of therapy cannot be defined in the same way as it might be when talking about recovery from a physical illness. Signs of anxiety will persist, and indeed anxiety is a normal human response, a part of living. For this reason, attention is most productively focused on recognizing and accepting anxiety, on handling its extreme manifestations, and on not letting it interfere with productive and satisfying ways of living. Such an attitude of acknowledgment and acceptance can have

---

Attending to the relationship

- Establishing a solid working alliance at the outset (or noting difficulties in doing so). Using active listening, accurate empathy, warmth, genuineness. Showing respect.
- Being sensitive to verbal and nonverbal signs of difficulty.
- Considering how to adapt to different needs, for example, for autonomy, or dependency.
- Being alert to one's own negative reactions (and seeking supervision).

Socializing people into the style of cognitive therapy

- Collaborative agenda setting, prioritizing, and using a clear, explicit rationale for specific interventions and assignments. Using guided discovery rather than lecturing, debate, or persuasion.
- Frequent two-way feedback, during and after sessions. Modeling openness and honesty.
- Welcoming the expression of doubts, criticisms, reservations.

Using practical methods

- Thorough assessment, including developing a sense of a patient's interpersonal style.
- Developing a shared problem formulation to provide a transparent overarching treatment rationale. Using this to develop clear, shared expectations of what therapy will involve (active collaboration, homework, etc.).
- Specification of agreed goals.
- Preparing the patient in advance for the possibility of difficulties, hiccups, setbacks, ups and downs in progress.
- Tape-recording sessions. Making time to listen and to reflect on difficulties.
- Encouraging patients to keep a "therapy notebook" in which they record their experiences of therapy (key observations, useful methods, moments of insight, new ideas, practical tips, etc.).

FIGURE 10.1. Guidelines for preventing problems in treatment process.

many subtle effects, such as reducing fear of anxiety itself, helping people to reflect more objectively on their experiences of it, reestablishing (when it is in doubt) the sense of being much like everyone else despite the anxiety, and so on. The explicit style of cognitive therapy, sensitively used, is invaluable as a tool for identifying and endorsing such attitudes, and an open discussion of these issues often contributes to developing self-confidence and self-worth, as it throws doubt on the assumptions that anxiety is a sign of weakness, abnormality, or poor worth, or evidence that confidence cannot grow (see also Chapter 8).

Practical guidelines for preventing and for managing problems that affect the course of treatment as a whole and on termination in particular are summarized in Figures 10.1 and 10.2. These guidelines exemplify important general aspects of cognitive therapy, and they are listed here because it is only too easy to forget them when difficulties or complications arise.

It is important to recognize that "ending treatment" usually starts long before the final session. At the very beginning of therapy—often in the very first session—a message about the process of change is more or less explicitly communicated to the patient. The essence of the message could be summarized as follows:

- Difficulties can be understood in terms of patterns of thinking, based on beliefs derived from experience, which influence emotion, body state, and behavior on a moment-to-moment basis.
- We will work together for a specified period (depending on the problem and on service constraints) to identify the specific patterns that are keeping the problem going, and to find alternatives to them.
- This means learning skills, and skills learning takes practice.
- For this reason, in addition to the work we do together, you will have opportunities to carry out homework assignments between sessions, practicing what you learn in your own setting.

Using the relationship

- Being alert to the emergence of difficulties, including nonverbal cues. Attending quickly to ruptures in the relationship, signs of disengagement, and so on.
- Taking care not to come across as judgmental, authoritarian, punitive, confrontational; maintaining an inquisitive, optimistic, problem-solving stance.
- Using empathy. Recognizing that people are usually "awkward" for good reason—if we saw things the way they do, we would have similar feelings and might behave in the same way.
- Being willing to recognize one's own contribution to difficulties, to investigate the thinking behind them, and to seek alternatives.

Using the style of cognitive therapy

- Being upfront (but not confrontational) about difficulties perceived.
- Using curiosity as a guiding principle—rather than defensiveness.
- Remaining collaborative ("Let's see what's going on here").
- Pinpointing the problem and using guided discovery to explore the thinking behind it, the feelings driving it, the elements of the formulation to which it relates, and so on.
- Adopting a participant-observer role, which recognizes that the therapist may be contributing to the difficulty, while helping both parties to decenter from it. Using what emerges to identify and to reexamine appraisals.

Using practical methods

- Sticking with the model: using the formulation and the methodology.
- Working with specifics, not just with broad generalities; linking work on beliefs and behaviors.
- Investigating how far what has happened in therapy might be relevant to difficulties elsewhere and, if so, helping the patient to generalize from what has been learned.
- Avoiding stereotyping, labeling, pathologizing (e.g., "resistant," "manipulative," "She must want to be like this," "He doesn't really want to change").
- Using consultation/supervision, especially if therapists' buttons have been pressed or they have encountered one of their own bugbears or blind spots.
- Toward the end of therapy, planning posttreatment contact ("booster" sessions, telephone contact, follow-up assessments, etc.).

FIGURE 10.2. Guidelines for resolving problems in treatment process.

- In the long run, the aim is to reach the point where I am irrelevant to you—you have learned how to resolve difficulties yourself, even new ones that you have not encountered before.
- After therapy, however, it is not realistic to expect that you will never have a moment's difficulty or distress, ever again—life is not like that.
- But, you will have a better idea of what to do about it when it happens.
- So sessions can be seen in a sense as training or coaching sessions—a chance to investigate problems and potential solutions, which you can then try out for yourself and discuss when we next meet—so that over time, you build up the knowledge and skills you need.

A helpful analogy is driving lessons: When the lessons stop, driving does not come to an end—rather, independent driving begins.

Similarly, preparation for ending treatment continues more or less explicitly from session to session. Summarizing key learning points, ensuring that new ideas are tried out in practice, relating what has been learned to the bigger picture (the case formulation), and so forth all contribute to a gradual transmission of knowledge, skills, and a general attitude to the uncertainty that brings anxiety with it, and to the meaning of having recurrent problems and difficulties. Guided discovery is central to this process, in terms of sharing responsibility for the work of therapy, and in terms of ensuring that learning is consolidated and rehearsed. Examples of helpful questions can be found in Figure 10.3.

Sharing responsibility with the patient (highlighting resources)

- What are your goals? How would you like things to be different?
- What shall we work on first?
- What's the next problem to tackle?
- How are you going to go about that?
- How might you handle that differently? What other ways could you use?
- How have you overcome similar difficulties before?
- What have you already learned that might help with this?
- What else do we need to work on?

Consolidating learning

- What did you learn from that?
- Supposing a similar situation came up in the future, what could you do about it, using what you have discovered today?
- Where else could you apply this?
- What did you do that worked?
- How could you improve on that?
- How could you take that further?
- What's the next step?

FIGURE 10.3. Ending treatment: Questions facilitating collaboration.

Addressing Specific Concerns

The specific concerns about treatment termination that emerge in relation to particular patients should be understandable in terms of the overall case formulation, as the following brief vignettes illustrate.

> Sally had always doubted her capacity to manage her life effectively. In treatment, she described a consistent pattern of relying on others to solve problems for her and shield her from anything that might cause her to become anxious or stressed. This pattern resulted from her parents' well-intentioned overprotectiveness. She was an immensely precious late child, and they had always done everything they could to keep her from harm and to help and support her. Consequently she never developed confidence that the world was (generally speaking) a safe place, and that she had the capacity within herself to deal with difficulties independently. In therapy, she found it hard to engage in behavioral experiments outside the session, even though with the therapist present she was able to take risks. She tended to answer "I don't know" when asked open questions, in case her answer was wrong, and frequently sought reassurance. She found it hard to see the point of treatment and repeatedly considered dropping out of therapy altogether, even when things seemed to be going well, predicting that it would all fall apart once she no longer had the therapist to rely on. Her preoccupation ("How many more sessions have we got left?") sometimes occupied center stage so completely that it was virtually impossible to proceed.

> Hugh, on the other hand, had no doubts about his capacity to manage difficulty and stress on his own. He had learned very early in life to be independent, to put others first (initially, his alcoholic mother), and to ignore his own needs and emotions. Ashamed of his home situation, he had learned to keep his problems to himself, suppress his feelings, and soldier on no matter how hard it was. Subsequently he found close relationships extremely hard, unless he could adopt a caring role. Therapy provided Hugh with a new and foreign experience: being on the receiving end of care, attention, and interest. He came to see the therapist as a close friend and ally, the only person with whom he could express his uncertainties and be himself. As the end of sessions approached, he became increasingly sad. Where would he ever be able to find kindness, help, and support for himself in the outside world?

Patients may openly communicate concerns like these, or they may leak out (in Hugh's case, e.g., looking tearful when the end of therapy was mentioned). Some, especially those who are anxious about displeasing others, try hard to hide their feelings. So it is important for therapists to bring up the issue themselves well before the end of the agreed sessions, for example, when giving and getting feedback on the work. Periodic therapy reviews (e.g., halfway through a planned course of sessions) also provide a context in which this can be done readily. When difficulties and complications have led to treatment being extended, it is important to schedule regular reviews, and repeatedly to raise the issue of ending treatment (e.g., "How will you use that idea later, when we are no longer meeting?"), so as to ensure that neither patient nor therapist develops the assumption that treatment *should* continue until all problems are solved.

Discussion about ending might start with a general comment and question: "People quite often have concerns about what will happen when treatment ends, wondering how things will go then. How do you feel about ending our work together? Is there anything you are concerned about?" As in the two cases above, the formulation often provides clues as to what concerns a particular person might have and suggests more specific inquiries, for example: "I know that you have often felt frightened of being abandoned by people—does that come up at all when we talk about ending our sessions?" The therapist should also be alert to nonverbal signals and, with sensitivity, follow them up, for example: "I noticed that you looked away when I said we had x sessions to go. Can you tell me what went through your mind just then?" The aim is to provide an opening for exploring the specific nature of patients' thinking about termination, and the impact this is having on their feelings and behavior in and between sessions. The standard change methods of cognitive therapy can then be brought to bear (questioning thoughts, seeking alternatives, behavioral experiments, imagery work, formulating and operating from new assumptions and beliefs, etc.). This transition will go more smoothly when patients have already acquired some of these skills, and are in a better position to collaborate on dealing with the issues.

> For example, it was not hard for Sally and her therapist to recognize that her fears mapped on to fears that she had felt for a long time, and in many situations. They worked on tentatively formulating an alternative belief about herself ("I can't cope" →"I am strong enough to manage"), and then collecting evidence consistent with it, day by day and week by week ("positive data logging"; Padesky, 1994). This included keeping a record of the between-session assignments that Sally carried out on her own, especially those that required her to think on her feet and adapt to changing circumstances (she saw this as an important part of strength). At the same time, the therapist was careful to minimize advice and suggestions, even when Sally demanded them, while relating what she was doing quite explicitly to their joint project of investigating Sally's new idea about her self. Gradually she was able to recognize that, although her therapist's support and advice were valuable, she was better able to manage difficulties and carry things forward than she had supposed. This did not mean that she was entirely confident about ending treatment, but it put her in a better position to begin to reduce session frequency as the final sessions approached, and to use the gaps as a means of consolidating her sense of her own capacity to function independently, even when all was not going smoothly.

> With Hugh, a different approach was necessary. His problem was in a sense the exact opposite of Sally's—if anything he was too independent. He found it difficult to be open enough about himself (especially his feelings) to be able to get close to others. So the therapist was filling a genuine gap, and it was important to acknowledge how important the relationship had been, how feeling sad about it coming to an end was natural, and how perhaps it had provided a model for future relationships that would allow Hugh to break down the wall he had built between himself and others. They worked together on identifying how people get close to one

another (e.g., mutual confidences, doing things together) and on questioning the patterns of thinking that made it difficult for Hugh to follow these steps, even supposing he knew what they were. This work paved the way for a series of behavioral experiments, not only on establishing and nourishing new relationships, but also on developing the ones he already had.

In Figure 10.4, readers will find a sequence of questions designed to help them to think through issues concerning treatment termination in relation to specific patients. This provides a framework for thinking around the problem, illuminating issues, and beginning the process of preparing for the end.

Preparing for the Future: "Therapy Blueprints"

Marlatt and Gordon (1985) used the metaphor of a journey to describe the patient's progress once treatment has ended. The therapist has been present as a guide and companion during the first stage of the journey, but now the patient must set off alone. Journeys involve pleasant landscapes and lovely views—but they also include precipices, dodgy corners, dark woods, swamps, rocky patches, and points at which it may be difficult to choose between alternative routes, and wrong turnings may be taken. So travelers would do well to provide themselves with resources—maps, equipment, nourishment, and the like—in the interests of staying on the paths that lead to their goals.

The "therapy blueprint" is designed to provide just such a resource. The objective is to consolidate new learning and lay the foundations for extending it so that patients are in a good position to deal with future setbacks and difficulties and to continue to develop as their own cognitive therapists. The resulting document can be thought of as a blueprint for the future. An illustrative example will be found in Figure 10.5.

A Possible Framework for Developing a Blueprint

There is no "right way" to construct a blueprint, but a helpful sequence of questions that readers might like to experiment with when approaching the end of therapy with their patients follows. The questions are addressed to the patient:

- How did my problems develop? (formative experiences, resultant beliefs and assumptions, events preceding onset, or triggering episodes of distress)
- What kept them going? (maintaining factors including patterns of thought, characteristic emotions, unhelpful behaviors, for example, safety-seeking behaviors, environmental factors—including if appropriate the broad social, cultural, and political context as well as ongoing adversity and negative life events, interpersonal factors)
- What did I learn in therapy that helped? (ideas, methods)
- What were my most unhelpful thoughts, assumptions, and beliefs? What alternatives did I find to them? (This can be summarized in two vertical columns.)
- How can I build on what I learned? (action planning, carrying new learning into my own life, consolidating/extending new skills, addressing outstanding issues, applying what I have learned to new areas, etc.)

Bring to mind a particular patient, with whom you are close to ending therapy. Call up a visual image of that person, the sound of his or her voice. Recall what your sessions have focused on, and any difficulties that have occurred in the therapeutic process. Remember the formulation (draw it out if you wish): key formative experiences; beliefs about self, world, and others; unhelpful assumptions; triggers for distress; the specific patterns of thinking, feeling, and behaving that maintain the problem. Take time to reflect on the answer to these questions, in relation to that particular patient. Make notes if you wish.

What is the importance of addressing termination with this particular person?

What problems may arise if you fail to do so?

When should you start ending treatment? (you may already have done so)

What do you intend to cover before finishing? Are you and the patient agreed on this?

What are your criteria for deciding to stop? And the patient's criteria?

How will you elicit concerns about termination?

What concerns might you expect your patient to have, given what you know about them?

How will you both go about working with those concerns?

What has already been done that will help? What knowledge and skills can the patient apply in this new area?

What do you expect of the patient during the follow-up period (e.g., systematically or informally continuing the work begun in therapy)?

What will you, the therapist, offer during the follow-up period (e.g., regular booster sessions, occasional/at need consultations, telephone or e-mail contact)?

What have you done to ensure that new learning has been consolidated and will be recalled and used by the patient when treatment ends?

FIGURE 10.4. Ending treatment: Questions for therapists.

How did my problems develop?

When I was young, my parents were very strict and bullying. They wanted me to be a success in life, but unfortunately what they did had the opposite effect. I became more and more self-conscious and unconfident and confused. I could see no way out of my difficulties, and so they came to contaminate my whole life. I thought I was useless and expected the worst of other people. So I took every opportunity to avoid challenges and kept away from people as much as I could. That was the only way I felt safe.

What kept them going?

I got into a negative spiral—my fears about coming out of my shell were so strong they made me avoid things more and more, and the more I avoided things, the more convinced I was that I was useless and life was passing me by. I had tons of rules and regulations about how I must behave and these added to the pressure. I never had a chance to find out if other people were actually like my parents—I just assumed they would be.

What did I learn in therapy that helped?

I have learned to take risks—or at least to recognize when I'm avoiding them, and what safety-seeking behaviors I'm using. I have learned to like myself more and appreciate that I am likeable. So I am starting to feel better about myself. I've reversed the spiral—good things feed into more good things. I have discovered that things are often not as bad in reality as they are in my imagination, and that even if I'm terrified at first, it gets easier. I have learned that it's no big deal to be shy—other people feel that way too.

What were my most unhelpful thoughts, assumptions, and beliefs?
What alternatives did I find to them?

If people notice I'm unconfident, they will not like or respect me. I know from experience that this is not true. I like and respect unconfident people, and so do others. It takes courage to be unconfident! *People are out to judge me.* Some people are like that, but most people are more concerned with being liked themselves and wanting to be nice and get to know people, not sitting in judgment on them. *I am unworthy.* This is simply not true. There are lots of reasons why I am worthy. I care about others and try not to hurt them. I am patient and understanding. I make a contribution to my community—I support local charities, for example, and do volunteer work. I make a stand on things I believe in. I help other people when I can. I am making the effort to confront my difficulties, even though it's hard.

How can I build on what I learned?

By carrying on with experiments, day by day, reviewing how I am doing and where I want to go next. Keep testing predictions, pushing back the boundaries, and make sure I'm not falling back into using safety-seeking behaviors. Keep recording good things about me. Keep reading my handouts and reminding myself what I've learned. Zap my negative thoughts. When I start blaming myself, stand back and look at the bigger picture—responsibility is usually shared, and it may be nothing to do with me. Remember panic attacks are just bodily sensations, that's all—nothing ever happens.

(continued)

FIGURE 10.5. Therapy blueprint: An illustrative example.

What will help me to do this?

Being clear what my goals are. Noticing how, the better I am, the more I can do for others. Keeping my partner up-to-date on what I'm doing. Rewarding myself when I take a step forward.

What will get in my way?

If I'm not well, or under pressure, then it's harder to keep moving on. Also if I spend time with my parents, they still tend to undermine me.

How can I tackle these barriers?

Be kind to myself if I'm under pressure or stressed or ill—looking after myself is part of feeling worthy. I can get back to taking things forward when I'm better. Don't spend too much time with my parents, and when I'm there, practice answering back to the negative things they say, even if it's only in my head. Talk it over when I get home, to get perspective.

What might lead to a setback for me?

As above—stress, pressure, illness, too much time with my parents. Plus if I have a setback to my plans such as not getting a job I want. Or if someone really doesn't seem to like or respect me—hard to remember that's just their opinion.

What cues will tell me I am having a setback?
What is my unique relapse signature?

Stomach upset. Being tempted to start drinking too much (or doing it). Wanting to shut myself away in my room and not see anyone.

What will I do once I notice the cues?

Take time out to relax and work out what is going on. Go over my notes and remind myself what I have learned and what I need to do. Do it. Don't keep it to myself—ask for help from my partner, or my family doctor if I need to, or telephone my therapist as she suggested, even though I think I should be able to manage alone by now. If I lose my way, a couple of sessions could be enough to get me going again.

FIGURE 10.5. (continued)

- What will help me to do this? (e.g., keeping my desired end point in mind, support, and encouragement from significant others)
- What will get in my way? (e.g., overconfidence, too much effort, don't want to think about it any more, other commitments and pressures) How can I tackle these barriers?
- What might lead to a setback for me? (e.g., future stresses, life problems, changes in circumstances or relationships, personal vulnerabilities such as predicating self-esteem on factors that cannot be controlled, such as employment or being loved)
- What cues will tell me I am having a setback? What is my unique relapse signature? (thoughts, feelings, body sensations, behavior, the behavior of others)
- What will I do once I notice the cues? (careful, detailed action plan)

These questions are intended to provide a space for reflection and for summarizing experiences of therapy and their implications, as well as for paying careful attention to possible future difficulties and how to deal with them. They make the assumption that, however successful treatment is, old patterns are never entirely deleted from the hard disk but, given the right access codes (experiences), will once again come on line. It may not be possible to stop this from happening, especially where the difficulties include strong elements of implicit memory (see Chapters 2 and 5), for example, in the context of traumatic or abusive past experiences. However, setbacks can be either magnified or nipped in the bud by the way patients respond to early warning signals. The blueprint is constructed to maximize the chances that their response will be something like, "Aha! Something here for me to attend to. Now, what do I need to do?" For this reason, it should be written down and kept somewhere easy to find, so that it can be readily consulted. It may be helpful for its location to be discussed with the therapist once it has been completed.

Therapist and patient can choose to work through the blueprint questions in session, or the patient can work on them as a homework assignment (or sequence of assignments) for subsequent in-session discussion. The therapist can use this as a valuable opportunity to review the therapy notes and make a note of ideas and interventions that seemed especially significant. The reason for this is that the patient may have a less complete record of therapy than the therapist and may toward the end of the encounter have forgotten methods used early on that were helpful at the time. The ideas of therapist and patient can then be integrated into the final version of the blueprint—always assuming the patient agrees with the therapist's observations. In a sense there is no "final version," given that it is not possible to predict everything that might arise. A blueprint should be seen as the best draft possible in the current state of knowledge, but never complete or covering every eventuality. Setbacks and difficulties can then be used as part of the learning process, which among other things helps to stimulate curiosity and problem solving, rather than despair, when they occur. So, for example, it is best to complete the draft before booster sessions, or before extending the interval between sessions as therapy draws to a close. In this way the patient has an opportunity to road test it repeatedly, identifying its shortcomings and weaknesses, and updating it accordingly.

Using Metaphors and Stories

Not all patients coming to the end of a course of cognitive therapy are able or willing to generate a detailed "blueprint" of the type described above. For example, if there have been problems in the therapy relationship, or in adjusting to the processes of therapy, these may reemerge as termination approaches. Just as metaphors can be used to convey metamessages near the start of therapy (see Chapters 3 and 4) they can be used with a similar purpose once the end point is in sight.

Judith's anxieties were accompanied by features of borderline personality disorder. Although therapy was largely successful in helping her to overcome her difficulties, she was still prone to "black-and-white thinking" and fears of abandonment. As her last session approached she compared her therapist to the parents of Hansel and Gretel, who repeatedly left the children in the forest, hoping that they would not find their way home. The patient had referred to this story earlier, comparing the therapist to the witch, whose sugar house looked attractive, but who (having lured the children there) intended to fatten them up, push them into the oven, and eat them. Rather than challenge this perspective through verbal discussion the therapist decided to counter it by using another story.

Pinkola Estes (1992) offered a collection of fairy stories for use in therapy. The therapist selected *Vasalisa*, a Russian version of the Cinderella story. Before her death Vasalisa's mother explains that although she will no longer be with her, she will give her a special doll that possesses intuition. When she is in trouble the doll will give her signs as to what she should or should not do. Vasalisa has a difficult life after her mother dies. Eventually her stepmother and stepsisters tell her that she must go to Baba Yaga's house to fetch fire for their home. The doll provides guidance throughout this difficult adventure, indicating how Vasalisa should act to escape danger. She returns with fire in a skull on a stick, and her stepmother and stepsisters turn to ashes on her return.

This story was presented to Judith as a metaphor for all she had learned in therapy, about being self-sufficient, and cultivating her own skills. At first she felt the story was a stupid one, but then she dreamed that she was coping on a long and difficult journey on her own, and she took away a copy of the story, accompanied by notes of what she had learned in therapy.

A PERSONAL BLUEPRINT
FOR TREATING ANXIETY DISORDERS

In this book, we have addressed many issues that face the practicing clinician when using cognitive therapy to treat some of the more complicated anxiety disorders. We reviewed the state of the art and summarized the central features of contemporary models and treatment protocols for anxiety disorders. We emphasized the central role of case formulation in making sense of patients' difficulties, especially where problems are long-standing, complex, and comorbid. We explored the value of encouraging metacognitive awareness, helping patients to change their relationship to their own thoughts and feelings so that they come to see these as passing mental and physical events, in which they can choose not to engage. We mapped the in-depth investigation of problematic cognitions, including images and memories, and described how to work with them. We examined the role of experiential learning through behavioral experiments. We focused on problems associated with low self-esteem and avoidance of affect and investigated the contribution of intolerance of uncertainty to anxiety. Finally, we explored how therapist and patient can address issues related to ending treatment and prepare for the future.

We end by suggesting a framework for reflecting on the parts of this book that you have read, so as to draw up your own "blueprint for the future." In Figure 10.6, you will find a sequence of questions to ask yourself, if you wish, to help to consolidate what you have learned and consider how you might carry your learning forward in your clinical work.

What were my goals in reading this book? What did I hope to find out? What questions did I want to answer? What knowledge and skills did I hope to acquire?

What progress have I made in relation to my goals? What have I learned? (Look back over what you have read and, if you can, bring to mind your thoughts about it.)

How can I carry forward what I have learned? What are my goals now? (e.g., further reading, discussion with colleagues, related workshops and training events, applying the ideas with patients). If I intend to apply the ideas with patients, then exactly who? And when?

What will help me to achieve my goals? How can I make the most of these things?

What will make it difficult for me to achieve my goals? How will I overcome the difficulties?

FIGURE 10.6. A personal blueprint.

References

Alloy, L. B., Abramson, L. Y., Gibb, B. E., Crossfield, A. G., Pieracci, A. M., Spasojevic, J., et al., (2004). Developmental antecedents of cognitive vulnerability to depression: Review of findings from the cognitive vulnerability to depression project. *Journal of Cognitive Psychotherapy, 18*, 115–133.

American Psychiatric Association. (2000). *Diagnostic and statistical manual of mental disorders* (4th ed., text rev.). Washington, DC: Author.

Arntz, A., & Weertman, A. (1999). Treatment of childhood memories: Theory and practice. *Behaviour Research and Therapy, 37*, 715–740.

Baer, R. A. (2003). Mindfulness training as a clinical intervention: A conceptual and empirical review. *Clinical Psychology: Science and Practice, 10*, 125–140.

Barlow, D. H. (1988). *Anxiety and its disorders: The nature and treatment of anxiety and panic.* New York: Guilford Press.

Barlow, D. H. (2002). *Anxiety and its disorders: The nature and treatment of anxiety and panic* (2nd ed.). New York: Guilford Press.

Barlow, D. H., Craske, M. G., Cerny, J. A., & Klosko, J. S. (1989). Behavioral treatment of panic disorder. *Behavior Therapy, 20*, 261–282.

Barnard, P., & Teasdale, J. D. (1991). Interacting cognitive subsystems: A systematic approach to cognitive-affective interaction and change. *Cognition and Emotion, 5*, 1–39.

Bateman, A. (2000). Integrative developments. *Psychotherapy Section Newsletter, 27*, 12–24.

Bateman, A., & Fonagy, P. (2004). *Psychotherapy for borderline personality disorder: Mentalization based treatment.* Oxford, UK: Oxford University Press.

Beard, C., & Wilson, J. P. (2002). *The power of experiential learning: A handbook for trainers and educators.* London: Kogan Page.

Beck, A. T. (1976). *Cognitive therapy and the emotional disorders.* New York: International Universities Press.

Beck, A. T., Emery, G., & Greenberg, R. (1985). *Anxiety disorders and phobias: A cognitive perspective.* New York: Basic Books.

Beck, A. T., Freeman, A., & Associates. (1990). *Cognitive therapy of personality disorders.* New York: Guilford Press.

Beck, A. T., Freeman A., Davis, D. D., & Associates. (2004). *Cognitive therapy of personality disorders* (2nd ed.). New York: Guilford Press.

Beck, A. T., & Hurvich, M. S. (1959). Psychological correlates of depression: I. Frequency of "masochistic" dream content in a private practice sample. *Psychosomatic Medicine, 21*, 50–55.

Beck, A. T., Rush, A. J., Shaw, B. F., & Emery, G. (1979). *Cognitive therapy of depression.* New York: Guilford Press.

Beck, A. T., & Ward, C. H. (1961). Dreams of depressed patients: Characteristic themes in manifest content. *Archives of General Psychiatry, 5*, 462–467.

Beck, J. S. (1995). *Cognitive therapy: Basics and beyond.* New York: Guilford Press.

Beck, J. S. (2005). *Cognitive therapy for challenging problems: What to do when the basics don't work.* New York: Guilford Press.

Beitman, B. D. (1992). Integration through fundamental similarities and useful differences among the schools. In J. C. Norcross & M. R Goldfried (Eds.), *Handbook of psychotherapy integration* (pp. 202–230). New York: Basic Books.

Bennett-Levy, J. (2006). Therapist skills: A cognitive model of their acquisition and refinement. *Behavioural and Cognitive Psychotherapy, 34*, 57–78.

Bennett-Levy, J., Butler, G., Fennell, M., Hackmann, A., Mueller, M., & Westbrook, D. (Eds.). (2004). *Oxford guide to behavioural experiments in cognitive therapy.* Oxford, UK: Oxford University Press.

Bennett-Levy, J., & Thwaites, R. (2007). Self and self-reflection in the therapeutic relationship: A conceptual map and practical strategies for the training, supervision and self-supervision of interpersonal skills. In P. Gilbert & R. L. Leahy (Eds.), *The therapeutic relationship in the cognitive-behavioral psychotherapies* (pp. 255–281). New York: Routledge.

Bennett-Levy, J., Westbrook, D., Fennell, M., Cooper, M., Rouf, K., & Hackmann, A. (2004). Behaviour experiments: Historical and conceptual underpinnings. In J. Bennett-Levy, G. Butler, M. Fennell, A. Hackmann, M. Mueller, & D. Westbrook (Eds.), *Oxford guide to behavioural experiments in cognitive therapy* (pp. 1–20). Oxford, UK: Oxford University Press.

Bieling, P. J., & Kuyken, W. (2003). Is cognitive case formulation science or science fiction? *Clinical Psychology: Science and Practice, 10*, 52–69.

Borkovec, T. D. (1994). The nature, functions and origins of worry. In G. C. L. Davey & F. Tallis (Eds.), *Worrying: Perspectives in theory, assessment, and treatment* (pp. 5–34). New York: Wiley.

Borkovec, T. D. (2004, September). *Generalised anxiety disorder.* Keynote address, EABCT Annual Conference, Manchester, UK.

Borkovec, T. D. (2007, July 16–17). *Interpersonal and experiential therapies for generalised anxiety disorder and their integration into CBT.* Oxford Cognitive Therapy Centre Workshop, Oxford, UK.

Borkovec, T. D., Alcaine, O. M., & Behar, E. (2004). Avoidance theory of worry and generalized anxiety disorder. In R. G. Heimberg, C. L. Turk, & D. S. Mennin (Eds.), *Generalized anxiety disorder: Advances in research and practice* (pp. 77–108). New York: Guilford Press.

Borkovec, T. D., Lyonfields, J. D., Wiser, S. L., & Deihl, L. (1993). The role of worrisome thinking in the supression of cardiovascular response to phobic imagery. *Behaviour Research and Therapy, 31*, 321–324.

Borkovec, T. D., & Newman, M. G. (1998). Worry and generalised anxiety disorder. In P. Salkovskis (Ed.), *Comprehensive clinical psychology* (Vol. 6, pp. 439–459). Oxford, UK: Elsevier.

Borkovec, T. D., & Whisman, M. A. (1996). Psychosocial treatment for generalized anxiety disorder. In M. R. Mavissakalian & R. F. Prien (Eds.), *Long-term treatments of anxiety disorders* (pp. 171–199). Washington, DC: American Psychiatric Press.

Brewin, C. R. (1997). Psychological defences and the distortion of meaning. In M. Power & C. R. Brewin (Eds.), *The transformation of meaning in psychological therapies* (pp. 107–123). Chichester, UK: Wiley.

Brewin, C. R. (2001). A cognitive neuroscience account of posttraumatic stress disorder and its treatment. *Behaviour Research and Therapy, 39*, 373–393.

Brewin, C. R., Dalgleish, T., & Joseph, S. (1996). A dual-representation theory of posttraumatic stress disorder. *Psychology Review, 103*, 670–686.

Brewin, C. R., & Lennard, H. (1999). Effects of mode of writing on emotional memories. *Journal of Traumatic Stress, 12*, 355–361.

Burns, D. D. (1980). *Feeling good.* New York: Avon Books.

Butler, G. (1998). Clinical formulation. In A. S. Bellack & M. Hersen (Eds.), *Comprehensive clinical psychology* (Vol. 6, pp. 1–24). Oxford, UK: Elsevier.

Butler, G. (1999a). Formulating meanings: Integration from the perspective of a cognitive therapist. *Psychotherapy Section Newsletter, 27*, 25–46.

Butler, G. (1999b). *Overcoming social anxiety and shyness.* London: Robinson.

Butler, G. (2006). The value of formulation: A question for debate. *Clinical Psychology Forum, 160*, 9–12.

Butler, G., & Anastasiades, P. (1988). Predicting response to anxiety management in patients with GAD. *Behaviour Research and Therapy, 26*, 531–534.

Butler, G., Fennell, M., Robson, P., & Gelder, M. (1991). A comparison of behavior therapy and cognitive behavior therapy in the treatment of generalized anxiety disorder. *Journal of Consulting and Clinical Psychology, 59*, 167–175.

Butler, G., & Hackmann, A. (2004). Social anxiety. In J. Bennett-Levy, G. Butler, M. Fennell, A. Hackmann, M. Mueller, & D. Westbrook (Eds.), *Oxford guide to behavioural experiments in cognitive therapy* (pp. 141–158). Oxford, UK: Oxford University Press.

Butler, G., & Holmes, E. (in press). Imagery and the self following childhood trauma: Observations concerning the use of drawings and external images. In L. Stopa (Ed.), *Imagery and the damaged self: Perspectives on imagery in cognitive therapy.* London: Routledge.

Butler, G., & Hope, T. (2007). *Manage your mind: The mental fitness guide.* Oxford, UK: Oxford University Press.

Butler, G., & Mathews, A. (1983). Cognitive processes in anxiety. *Advances in Behaviour Therapy and Research, 5*, 51–62.

Butler, G., & Rouf, K. (2004). Generalized anxiety disorder. In J. Bennett-Levy, G. Butler, M. Fennell, A. Hackmann, M. Mueller, & D. Westbrook (Eds.), *Oxford guide to behavioural experiments in cognitive therapy* (pp. 121–137). Oxford, UK: Oxford University Press.

Butler, G., & Surawy, C. (2004). Avoidance of affect. In J. Bennett-Levy, G. Butler, M. Fennell, A. Hackmann, M. Mueller, & D. Westbrook (Eds.), *Oxford guide to behavioural experiments in cognitive therapy* (pp. 351–369). Oxford, UK: Oxford University Press.

Butler, G., Wells, A., & Dewick, H. (1995). Differential effect of worry and imagery after exposure to stressful stimulus. *Behavioural and Cognitive Psychotherapy, 25*, 45–56.

Cellucci, A. J., & Lawrence, P. S. (1978). Individual

differences in self-reported sleep variable correlations among nightmare sufferers. *Journal of Clinical Psychology, 34*, 721–725.

Chadwick, P. D., Birchwood, M. J., & Trower, P. (1996). *Cognitive therapy for delusions, voices and paranoia.* Chichester, UK: Wiley.

Chambless, D. L., & Goldstein, A. J. (1982). *Agoraphobia: Multiple perspectives on theory and treatment.* New York: Wiley.

Clark, D. A., & Beck, A. T. (1999). *Scientific foundations of cognitive theory and therapy of depression.* New York: Wiley.

Clark, D. M. (1986). A cognitive approach to panic. *Behaviour Research and Therapy, 24*, 461–470.

Clark, D. M. (1988). A cognitive model of panic attacks. In S. Rachman & J. Maser (Eds.), *Panic: Psychological perspectives* (pp. 121–132). Hillsdale, NJ: Erlbaum.

Clark, D. M. (1989). Anxiety states: Panic and generalised anxiety. In K. Hawton, P. M. Salkovskis, J. Kirk, & D. M. Clark (Eds.), *Cognitive behaviour therapy for psychiatric problems: A practical guide* (pp. 52–96). Oxford, UK: Oxford University Press.

Clark, D. M. (1999). Anxiety disorders: Why they persist and how to treat them. *Behaviour Research and Therapy, 37*, S5–S27.

Clark, D. M. (2004). Developing new treatments: On the interplay between theories, experimental science and clinical innovation. *Behaviour Research and Therapy, 429*, 1089–1104.

Clark, D. M., Ehlers, A., Hackmann, A., McManus, F., Fennell, M., Grey, N., et al. (2006). Cognitive therapy versus exposure and applied relaxation in social phobia: A randomized controlled trial. *Journal of Consulting and Clinical Psychology, 74*, 568–578.

Clark, D. M., Salkovskis, P. M., Hackmann, A., Middleton, H., Anastasiades, P., & Gelder, M. G. (1994). A comparison of cognitive therapy, applied relaxation and imipramine in the treatment of panic disorder. *British Journal of Psychiatry, 164*, 759–769.

Clark, D. M., Salkovskis, P. M., Hackmann, A., Wells, A., Ludgate, J., & Gelder, M. (1999). Brief cognitive therapy for panic disorder: A randomized controlled trial. *Journal of Consulting and Clinical Psychology, 67*, 583–589.

Clark, D. M., & Wells, A. (1995). The cognitive model of social phobia. In R. G. Heimberg, M. R. Liebowitz, D. A. Hope, & F. R. Schneier (Eds.), *Social phobia: Diagnosis, assessment and treatment* (pp. 69–93). New York: Guilford Press.

Conway, M. A., Meares, K., & Standart, S. (2004). Images and goals. *Memory, 12*, 525–531.

Craske, M. G., Farchione, T., Tsao, J., & Mystkowski, J. (1998, September). *Comorbidity and panic disorder.* Paper presented at the EABCT annual conference, Madrid, Spain.

Dalgleish, T., & Power, M. (Eds.). (1999). *Handbook of cognition and emotion.* Chichester, UK: Wiley.

Davey, G., & Tallis, F. (Eds.). (1994). *Worrying: Perspectives on theory, assessment and treatment.* Chichester, UK: Wiley.

Day, S., Holmes, E. M., & Hackmann, A. (2004). Occurrence of imagery and its links to memory in agoraphobia. *Memory, 12*, 525–531.

de Silva, P., & Marks, M. (1999). The role of traumatic experiences in the genesis of obsessive-compulsive disorder. *Behaviour Research and Therapy, 37*, 941–951.

Dugas, M. J., Gagnon, F., Ladouceur, R., & Freeston, M. H. (1998). Generalized anxiety disorder: A preliminary test of a conceptual model. *Behaviour Research and Therapy, 36*, 215–226.

Dugas, M. J., Ladouceur, R., Leger, E., Freeson, M., Langlois, F., Provencher, M. D., et al. (2003). Group cognitive-behavioral therapy for generalized anxiety disorder: Treatment outcome and long-term follow-up. *Journal of Consulting and Clinical Psychology, 71*, 821–825.

Dugas, M. J., Letarte, H., Rheaume, J., Freeston, M., & Ladouceur, R. (1995). Worry and problem solving: Evidence of a special relationship. *Cognitive Therapy and Research, 19*, 109–120.

Edwards, D. (1989). Cognitive restructuring through guided imagery. Lessons from gestalt therapy. In A. Freeman, K. M. Simon, L. E. Beutler, & H. Arkowitz (Eds.), *Comprehensive handbook of cognitive therapy* (pp. 283–297). New York: Plenum Press.

Edwards, D. (1990). Cognitive therapy and the restructuring of early memories through guided imagery. *Journal of Cognitive Psychotherapy: An International Quarterly, 1*, 33–49.

Eells, T. D. (1997). *Handbook of psychotherapy case formulation.* New York: Guilford Press.

Eells, T. D. (2006). *Handbook of psychotherapy case formulation* (2nd ed.). New York: Guilford Press.

Eells, T. D., Kendjelic, E. M., & Lucas, C. P (1998). What's in a case formulation? Development and use of a content coding manual. *Journal of Psychotherapy Practice and Research, 7*, 144–153.

Ehlers, A., & Clark, D. M. (2000). A cognitive model of persistent PTSD. *Behaviour Research and Therapy, 38*, 319–345.

Ehlers, A., Clark, D. M., Hackmann, A., McManus, F., & Fennell, M. (2005). Cognitive therapy for posttraumatic stress disorder: Development and evaluation. *Behaviour Research and Therapy, 43*, 413–431.

Ehlers, A., Hackmann, A., & Michael, T. (2004). Intrusive re-experiencing in post-traumatic stress disorder: Phenomenology, theory, and therapy. *Memory, 12*, 403–415.

Ehlers, A., Hackmann, A., Steil, R., Clohessy, S., Wenninger, K., & Winter, H. (2002). The nature of intrusive memories after trauma: The warning signal hypothesis. *Behaviour Research and Therapy, 40*, 995–1002.

Engelkamp, J. (1998). *Memory for actions.* Hove, UK: Psychology Press.

Epstein, S. (1998). *Constructive thinking: The key to emotional intelligence.* Westport, CT: Praeger.

Fennell, M. J. V. (1997). Self-esteem: A cognitive perspective. *Behavioural and Cognitive Psychotherapy, 25,* 1–25.

Fennell, M. J. V. (1998). Low self-esteem. In N. Tarrier, A. Wells, & G. Haddock (Eds.), *Treating complex cases: The cognitive behavioural therapy approach* (pp. 217–240). Chichester, UK: Wiley.

Fennell, M. J. V. (1999). *Overcoming low self-esteem.* London: Constable-Robinson.

Fennell, M. J. V. (2004). Depression, low self-esteem and mindfulness. *Behaviour Research and Therapy, 42,* 1053–1067.

Fennell, M. J. V. (2006). *Overcoming low self-esteem self-help course: A 3-part programme based on cognitive behavioural techniques.* London: Constable-Robinson.

Fennell, M. J. V. (2007). Low self-esteem. In N. Kazantzis & L. L'Abate (Eds.), *Handbook of homework assignments in psychotherapy: Research, practice and prevention* (pp. 297–314). New York: Springer.

Foa, E. B., & Kozak, M. J. (1986). Emotional processing of fear: Exposure to corrective information. *Psychological Bulletin, 31,* 269–278.

Foa, E. B., Molnar, C., & Cashman, L. (1995). Change in rape narratives during exposure therapy for posttraumatic stress disorder. *Journal of Traumatic Stress, 8,* 675–690.

Foa, E. B., & Rothbaum, B. O. (1998). *Treating the trauma of rape: Cognitive-behavior therapy for PTSD.* New York: Guilford Press.

Fothergill, C. D., & Kuyken, W. (2003). Case formulation and treatment concepts among novice, experienced, and expert cognitive-behavioural and psychodynamic therapists. *Psychotherapy Research, 13,* 187–204.

Freeman, A. (1981). Dreams and images in cognitive therapy. In G. Emery, S. Hollon, & R. C. Bedrosian (Eds.), *New directions in cognitive therapy: A case book* (pp. 224–238). New York: Guilford Press.

Freeston, M., Rheaume, J., & Ladouceur, R. (1996). Correcting faulty appraisals of obsessive thoughts. *Behaviour Research and Therapy, 34,* 433–446.

Friedman, R. S., & Forster, J. (2001). The effects of promotion and prevention cues on creativity. *Journal of Personality and Social Psychology, 81,* 1001–1013.

Gendlin, E. T. (1996). *Focusing-oriented psychotherapy: A manual of the experiential method.* New York: Guilford Press

Gilbert, P. (Ed.). (2005a). *Compassion: Conceptualisations, research and use in psychotherapy.* London: Routledge.

Gilbert, P. (2005b). Compassion and cruelty: A biopsychosocial approach. In P. Gilbert (Ed.), *Compassion: Conceptualisations, research and use in psychotherapy* (pp. 9–74). London: Routledge.

Goldfried, M. R. (2004). Integrating integratively oriented brief psychotherapy. *Journal of Psychotherapy Integration, 14,* 93–105.

Goldstein, J., & Kornfield, J. (2001). *Seeking the heart of wisdom: The path of insight meditation.* Boston: Shambhala Classics.

Goleman, D. (1996). *Emotional intelligence.* London: Bloomsbury.

Greenberg, L. S., & Paivio, S. C. (1997). *Working with emotions in psychotherapy.* New York: Guilford Press.

Greenberger, D., & Padesky, C. A. (1995). *Mind over mood.* New York: Guilford Press.

Grey, N., Young, K., & Holmes, E. A. (2002). Cognitive restructuring within reliving: A treatment for peritraumatic emotional "hotspots" in posttraumatic stress disorder. *Behavioural and Cognitive Psychotherapy, 30,* 37–56.

Gross, J. J. (1998). The emerging field of emotion regulation: An integrative review. *Review of General Psychology, 2,* 271–299.

Gross, J. J. (Ed.). (2007). *Handbook of emotion regulation.* New York: Guilford Press.

Hackmann, A. (1998a). Cognitive therapy for panic and agoraphobia: Working with complex cases. In N. Tarrier, A. Wells, & G. Haddock (Eds.), *Treating complex cases: The cognitive behavioural approach* (pp. 27–43). Chichester, UK: Wiley.

Hackmann, A. (1998b). Working with images in clinical psychology. In A. Bellack & M. Hersen (Eds.), *Comprehensive clinical psychology* (Vol. 6, pp. 301–318). Oxford, UK: Elsevier.

Hackmann, A. (2005a). Compassionate imagery in the treatment of early memories in Axis I anxiety disorders. In P. Gilbert (Ed.), *Compassion: Conceptualisations, research and use in psychotherapy* (pp. 352–368). London: Brunner-Routledge.

Hackmann, A. (2005b, July). *Sleep and PTSD.* Paper presented at the 33rd annual conference of the British Association for Behavioural and Cognitive Psychotherapy, University of Canterbury, UK.

Hackmann, A., Clark, D., & McManus, F. (2000). Recurrent images and early memories in social phobia. *Behaviour Research and Therapy, 38,* 601–610.

Hackmann, A., & Holmes, E. A. (2004). Reflecting on imagery: A clinical perspective and overview of the special issue on mental imagery and memory in psychopathology. *Memory, 12,* 389–402.

Hackmann, A., Surawy, C., & Clark, D. M. (1998). Seeing yourself through other's eyes: A study of spontaneously occurring images in social phobia. *Behavioural and Cognitive Psychotherapy, 26,* 3–12.

Harvey, A. G., Clark, D. M., Ehlers, A., & Rapee, R. M. (2000). Social anxiety and self-impression: Cognitive preparation enhances the beneficial effects of video feedback following a stressful social task. *Behaviour Research and Therapy, 38,* 1183–1192.

Harvey, A., Watkins, E., Mansell, W., & Shafran, R. (2004). *Cognitive behavioural processes across psychological disorders*. Oxford, UK: Oxford University Press.

Hawton, K., Salkovskis, P. M., Kirk, J., & Clark, D. M. (1989). *Cognitive behaviour therapy for psychiatric problems*. Oxford, UK: Oxford University Press.

Hayes, S. C., Strosahl, K. D., & Wilson, K. G. (1999). *Acceptance and commitment therapy: An experiential approach to behaviour change*. New York: Guilford Press.

Hayes, S. C., Wilson, K. G., Strosahl, K., Gifford, E. V., & Follette, V. M. (1996). Experiential avoidance and behavioral disorders: A functional dimensional approach to diagnosis and treatment. *Journal of Consulting and Clinical Psychology, 64*, 1152–1168.

Heimberg, R. G., Turk, C. L., & Mennin, D. S. (2004). *Generalized anxiety disorder: Advances in research and practice*. New York: Guilford Press.

Hertel, P. T. (2002). Cognitive biases in anxiety and depression: Introduction to the special issue. *Cognition and Emotion, 16*, 321–330.

Hertel, P. T. (2004). Habits of thought produce memory biases in anxiety and depression. In J. Yiend (Ed.), *Cognition, emotion and psychopathology* (pp. 109–129). Cambridge, UK: Cambridge University Press.

Hodgson, R., & Rachman, S. J. (1974). Desynchrony in measures of fear. *Behaviour Research and Therapy, 12*, 319–326.

Hoffart, A., Hackmann, A., & Sexton, H. (2006). Interpersonal fears among patients with panic disorder with agoraphobia. *Behavioural and Cognitive Psychotherapy, 34*, 359–363.

Hoffman, E. (1989). *Lost in translation*. London: Minerva Press.

Holmes, E. A., & Hackmann, A. (Eds.). (2004). Mental imagery and memory in psychopathology [Special Issue]. *Memory, 12*(4).

James, I. A. (2001). Schema therapy: The next generation, but should it carry a health warning? *Behavioural and Cognitive Psychotherapy, 29*, 401–407.

Janoff-Bulman, R. (1992). *Shattered assumptions: Towards a new psychology of trauma*. New York: Free Press.

Jaycox, L. H. (1998). Post-traumatic stress disorder. In A. S. Bellack & M. Hersen (Eds.), *Comprehensive clinical psychology* (Vol. 6, pp. 499–518). Oxford, UK: Pergamon.

Johles, L. (2005, June 12–14). *How to use drawings within a CBT-framework*. Workshop presented at the annual conference of the European Association for Behavioural and Cognitive Therapies, Gothenberg, Sweden.

Johnstone, L. (2006). Controversies and debates about formulations. In L. Johnstone & R. Dallos (Eds.), *Formulation in psychology and psychotherapy* (pp. 208–235). London: Routledge.

Kellner, R., Neidhardt, J., Krakow, B., & Pathak, D.

(1992). Changes in chronic nightmares after one session of desensitization or rehearsal instructions. *American Journal of Psychiatry, 49*, 569–663.

Kessler, R. C., McGonagle, K. A., Zhao, S., Nelson, C. B., Hughes, M., Eshleman, S., et al. (1994). Lifetime and twelve month prevalence of DSM-III-R psychiatric disorders in the United States. *Archives of General Psychiatry, 51*, 8–19.

Kessler, R. C., Sonnega, A., Bromet, E., Hughes, M., & Nelson, C. B. (1995). Posttraumatic stress disorder in the National Comorbidity Survey. *Archives of General Psychiatry, 52*, 1048–1060.

Kirk, J., & Rouf, K. (2004). Specific phobias. In J. Bennett-Levy, G. Butler, M. Fennell, A. Hackmann, M. Mueller, & D. Westbrook (Eds.), *Oxford guide to behavioural experiments in cognitive therapy* (pp. 161–180). Oxford, UK: Oxford University Press.

Knowles, M. S. (1990). *The adult learner: A neglected species*. London: Gulf Publishing.

Knowles, M. S., Holton, E. F. III, & Swanson, R. A. (2005). *The adult learner: The definitive classic in adult education and human resource development*. Amsterdam, CA: Elsevier.

Kolb, D. A. (1984). *Experiential learning*. Englewood Cliffs, NJ: Prentice Hall.

Krakow, B., Kellner, R., Pathak, D., & Lambert, L. (1995). Imagery rehearsal treatment for chronic nightmares. *Behaviour Research and Therapy, 33*, 837–843.

Krakow, B., & Zadra, A. (2006). Clinical management of chronic nightmares: Imagery rehearsal therapy. *Behavioral Sleep Medicine, 4*, 45–70

Ladouceur, R., Dugas, M. J., Freeston, M. H., Leger, E., Gagnon, F., & Thibodeau, N. (2000). Efficacy of cognitive-behavioural therapy for generalized anxiety disorder: Evaluation in a controlled clinical trial. *Journal of Consulting and Clinical Psychology, 68*, 957–964.

Layden, M. A., Newman, C., Freeman, A., & Byers Morse, S. (1993). *Cognitive therapy of borderline personality disorder*. Boston: Allyn & Bacon.

Leahy, R. L. (2001). *Overcoming resistance in cognitive therapy*. New York: Guilford Press.

Leahy, R. L. (2002). A model of emotional schemas. *Cognitive and Behavioural Practice, 9*, 177–190.

Leahy, R. L. (2003). *Cognitive therapy techniques: A practitioner's guide*. New York: Guilford Press.

Leahy, R. L., & Hollon, S. J. (2000). *Treatment plans and interventions for depression and anxiety disorders*. New York: Guilford Press.

Lee, D. (2005). The perfect nurturer: A model to develop a compassionate mind within the context of cognitive therapy. In P. Gilbert (Ed.), *Compassion: Conceptualisations, research and use in psychotherapy* (pp. 326–351). London: Routledge.

Levis, D. J. (1980). Implementing the technique of implosive therapy. In A. Goldstein & E. B. Foa (Eds.), *Handbook of behavioral interventions* (pp. 92–151). New York: Wiley.

Linehan, M. M. (1993a). *Cognitive behavioral treatment of borderline personality disorder*. New York: Guilford Press.

Linehan, M. M. (1993b). *Skills training manual for treating borderline personality disorder*. New York: Guilford Press.

Ma, H., & Teasdale, J. D. (2004). Mindfulness-based cognitive therapy for depression: Replication and exploration of differential relapse prevention effects. *Journal of Consulting and Clinical Psychology, 72*, 31–40.

MacLeod, C. (1996). Anxiety and cognitive processes. In I. G. Sarason, B. P. Sarason, & G. R. Pierce (Eds.), *Cognitive interference: Theories, methods and findings* (pp. 47–76). Hillsdale, NJ: Erlbaum.

Mansell, W., & Clark, D. M. (1999). How do I appear to others? Social anxiety and processing of the observable self. *Behaviour Research and Therapy, 37*, 419–434.

Mansell, W., & Lam, D. (2004). A preliminary study of autobiographical memory in remitted bipolar and unipolar depression and the role of imagery in the specificity of memory. *Memory, 12*, 437–446.

Marks, I. M. (1978). Rehearsal relief of a nightmare. *British Journal of Psychiatry, 133*, 461–465.

Marlatt, G. A., & Gordon, J. R. (1985). *Relapse prevention: Maintenance strategies in the treatment of addictive behaviors*. New York: Guilford Press.

Mathews, A., & MacLeod, C. (2002). Induced processing biases have causal effects on anxiety. *Cognition and Emotion, 16*, 331–354.

Mayer, J. D., Salovey, P., Caruso, D. R., & Sitarenios, G. (2003). Measuring emotional intelligence with MSCEIT V2. *Emotion, 3*, 97–105.

Mineka, S., Walsh, D., & Clark, L. A. (1998). Comorbidity of anxiety and unipolar mood disorder. *Annual Review of Psychology, 49*, 377–412.

Mogg, K., & Bradley, B. P. (1998). A cognitive-motivational analysis of anxiety. *Behaviour Research and Therapy, 36*, 809–848.

Mogg, K., & Bradley, B. P. (2004). A cognitive-motivational perspective on the processing of threat information and anxiety. In J. Yiend (Ed.), *Cognition and emotion and psychopathology* (pp. 68–85). Cambridge, UK: Cambridge University Press.

Mooney, K. A., & Padesky, C. A. (2000). Applying client creativity to recurrent problems: Constructing possibilities and tolerating doubt. *Journal of Cognitive Psychotherapy, 14*, 149–161.

Moore, R. G. (1996). It's the thought that counts: The role of intentions and meta-awareness in cognitive therapy. *Journal of Cognitive Psychotherapy, 10*, 255–269.

Morrison, N., & Westbrook, D. (2004). Obsessive compulsive disorder. In J. Bennett-Levy, G. Butler, M. J. V. Fennell, A. Hackmann, M. Mueller, & D. Westbrook (Eds.), *Oxford guide to behavioural experiments in cognitive therapy* (pp. 101–118). Oxford, UK: Oxford University Press.

Newman, M. G., & Borkovec, T. D. (2002). Cognitive behavioural therapy for worry and generalised anxiety disorder. In G. Simos (Ed.), *Cognitive behaviour therapy, a guide for the practising clinician* (pp. 150–172). Sussex, UK: Brunner-Routledge.

Nezu, A. M., Nezu, C. M., & Lombardo, E. (2004). *Cognitive-behavioral case formulation and treatment design: A problem-solving approach*. New York: Springer.

Obsessive–Compulsive Cognitions Working Group. (1997). Cognitive assessment of obsessive-compulsive disorder. *Behaviour Research and Therapy, 35*, 667–681.

Ornstein, R. (1991). *The evolution of consiousness*. New York: Touchstone.

P. S. (2006). Commentary on "The value of formulation: A question for debate." *Clinical Psychology Forum, 160*, 13–14.

Ost, L. G. (1997). Rapid treatment of specific phobias. In G. C. L. Davey (Ed.), *Phobia: A handbook of theory, research and treatment* (pp. 227–246). Chichester, UK: Wiley.

Padesky, C. A. (1993a). Schema change as self-prejudice. *International Cognitive Therapy Newsletter, 5/6*, 16–17.

Padesky, C. A. (1993b, September 24). *Socratic questioning: Changing minds or guiding discovery?* Keynote address delivered at the European Congress of Behavioural and Cognitive Therapies, London. Available from *www.padesky. com*.

Padesky, C. A. (1994). Schema-change processes in cognitive therapy. *Clinical Psychology and Psychotherapy, 1*, 267–278.

Padesky, C. (1997). A more effective treatment focus for social phobia? *International Cognitive Therapy Newsletter, 11*, 1–3.

Padesky, C. A., & Beck, J. (2003). Avoidant personality disorder. In A. T. Beck, A. Freeman, D. D. Davis, & Associates (Eds.), *Cognitive therapy of personality disorders* (2nd ed., pp. 293–319). New York: Guilford Press.

Padesky, C. A., with Greenberger, D. (1995). *Clinician's guide to mind over mood*. New York: Guilford Press.

Panksepp, J. (2004). *Affective neuroscience: The foundations of human and animal emotions*. New York: Oxford University Press.

Persons, J. B. (1989). *Cognitive therapy in practice: A case-formulation approach*. New York: Norton.

Persons, J. B., & Bertagnolli, A. (1999). Inter-rater reliability of cognitive-behavioral case formulations of depression: A replication. *Cognitive Therapy and Research, 23*, 271–283.

Persons, J. B., Mooney, K. A., & Padesky, C. A. (1995). Inter-rater reliability of cognitive-behavioural case formulations. *Cognitive Therapy and Research, 19*, 21–34.

Pinel, E., & Constantino, M. J. (2003). Putting self

psychology to good use: When social and clinical psychologists unite. *Journal of Psychotherapy Integration, 13*, 9–32.

Power, M. J. (1997). Conscious and unconscious representations of meaning. In M. J. Power & C. R. Brewin (Eds.), *The transformation of meaning* (pp. 57–73). Chichester, UK: Wiley.

Power, M. J., & Dalgleish, T. (1997). *Cognition and emotion: From order to disorder*. Hove, UK: Psychology Press.

Pinkola Estes, C. (1992). *Women who run with the wolves: Myths and stories of the wild woman archetype*. New York: Ballantine Books.

Pratt, D., Cooper, M. J., & Hackmann, A. (2004). Imagery and its characteristics in people who are anxious about spiders. *Behavioural and Cognitive Psychotherapy, 32*(2), 165–176.

Rachman, S. J. (1980). Emotional processing. *Behaviour Research and Therapy, 18*, 51–60.

Rachman, S. J. (2001). Emotional processing, with special reference to post-traumatic stress disorder. *International Review of Psychiatry, 13*, 164–171.

Rachman, S. J., & Bichard, S. (1988). The overprediction of fear. *Clinical Psychology Review, 8*, 303–312.

Rapee, R. G., & Heimberg, R. H. (1997). A cognitive-behavioral approach to anxiety in social phobia. *Behaviour Research and Therapy, 35*, 741–756.

Roemer, L., Borkovec, T. D., Posa, S., & Lyonfields, J. (1991, November). *Generalized anxiety disorder in an analogue population: The role of past trauma*. Paper presented at the annual convention of the Association for the Advancement of Behavior Therapy, New York.

Rothschild, B. (2000). *The body remembers: The psychophysiology of trauma and trauma treatment*. New York: Norton.

Rouf, K., Fennell, M., Westbrook, D., Cooper, M., & Bennett-Levy, J. (2004). Devising effective behavioural experiments. In J. Bennett-Levy, G. Butler, M. Fennell, A. Hackmann, M. Mueller, & D. Westbrook (Eds.), *Oxford guide to behavioural experiments in cognitive therapy* (pp. 21–58). Oxford, UK: Oxford University Press.

Safran, J. D., & Muran, J. C. (2000). *Negotiating the therapeutic alliance: A relational treatment guide*. New York: Guilford Press.

Safran, J. D., & Segal, Z. V. (1990). *Interpersonal process in cognitive therapy*. Northvale, NJ: Jason Aronson.

Salkovskis, P. M. (1985). Obsessive-compulsive problems: A cognitive behavioural analysis. *Behaviour Research and Therapy, 23*, 571–583.

Salkovskis, P. M. (1991). The importance of behavior in the maintenance of anxiety and panic: a cognitive account. *Behavioural and Cognitive Psychotherapy, 19*, 6–19.

Salkovskis, P. M. (1996). The cognitive approach to anxiety: Threat beliefs, safety-seeking behavior, and the special case of health anxiety obses-

sions. In P. M. Salkovskis (Ed.), *Frontiers of cognitive therapy* (pp. 48–74). New York: Guilford Press.

Salkovskis, P. M. (1999). Understanding and treating obsessive-compulsive disorder. *Behaviour Research and Therapy, 37*, S29–S52.

Salkovskis, P. M., Clark, D. M., & Gelder, M. G. (1996). Cognition-behavior links in the persistence of panic. *Behaviour Research and Therapy, 34*, 453–458.

Salkovskis, P. M., Clark, D. M., Hackmann, A., Wells, A., & Gelder, M. G. (1999). An experimental investigation of the role of safety behaviours in the maintenance of panic disorder with agoraphobia. *Behaviour Research and Therapy, 37*, 559–574.

Salkovskis, P. M., Forrester, E., Richards, H. C., & Morrison, N. (1999). The devil is in the detail: Conceptualizing and treating obsessional problems. In N. Tarrier, A. Wells, & G. Haddock (Eds.), *Treating complex cases: The cognitive behavioural approach* (pp. 46–80). Chichester, UK: Wiley.

Salkovskis, P. M., & Hackmann, A. (1997). Agoraphobia. In G. Davey (Ed.), *Phobias: A handbook of theory, research and treatment* (pp. 27–62). Chichester, UK: Wiley.

Salkovskis, P. M., Hackmann, A., Wells, A., Gelder, M. G., & Clark, D. M. (2007). Belief disconfirmation versus habituation approaches to situational exposure in panic disorder with agoraphobia: A pilot study. *Behaviour Research and Therapy, 45*, 877–885.

Salkovskis, P. M., & Warwick, H. M. (1986). Morbid preoccupations, health anxiety and reassurance: A cognitive-behavioural approach to hypochondriasis. *Behaviour Research and Therapy, 2*, 597–602.

Schön, D. A. (1983). *The reflective practitioner: How professionals think in action*. New York: Basic Books.

Schön, D. A. (1987). *Educating the reflective practitioner: Towards a new design for teaching and learning in the professions*. San Francisco: Jossey-Bass.

Segal, Z. V., Williams, J. M. G., & Teasdale, J. D. (2002). *Mindfulness-based cognitive therapy for depression: A new approach to preventing relapse*. New York: Guilford Press.

Shafran, R., Thordarson, D. S., & Rachman, S. J. (1996). Thought-action fusion in obsessive-compulsive disorder. *Journal of Anxiety Disorders, 10*, 379–391.

Shapiro, F. (2001). *Eye movement desensitization and reprocessing (EMDR): Basic principles, protocols, and procedures*. New York: Guilford Press.

Silver, A., Sanders, D., Morrison, N., & Cowey, C. (2004). In J. Bennett-Levy, G. Butler, M. Fennell, A. Hackmann, M. Mueller, & D. Westbrook (Eds.), *Oxford guide to behavioural experiments in cognitive therapy* (pp. 81–98). Oxford, UK: Oxford University Press.

Simonton, D. K. (2005). Creativity. In C. R. Snyder

& S. J. Lopez (Eds.), *Handbook of positive psychology* (pp. 189–210). Oxford, UK: Oxford University Press.

Simos, G. (2002). *Cognitive behaviour therapy: A guide for the practising clinician*. Sussex, UK: Brunner-Routledge.

Smucker, M., Dancu, C., Foa, E., & Neideree, J. L. (1995). Imagery rescripting: A new treatment for survivors of childhood sexual abuse suffering from posttraumatic stress. *Journal of Cognitive Psychotherapy: An International Quarterly, 9*, 3–11.

Speckens, A., Hackmann, A., & Ehlers, A. (2003, July). *Imagery and early traumatic memories in obsessive-compulsive disorder*. Paper presented at the 31st annual conference of the British Association for Behavioural and Cognitive Psychotherapy, University of York, UK.

Stampfl, T., & Levis, D. J. (1967). Essentials of implosive therapy: A learning theory based psychodynamic behavioural therapy. *Journal of Abnormal Psychology, 72*, 496–503.

Sternberg, R. J. (Ed.). (1998). *The handbook of creativity*. Cambridge, UK: Cambridge University Press.

Tarrier, N. (2006). *Case formulation in cognitive behaviour therapy: The treatment of challenging and complex cases*. Sussex, UK: Routledge.

Teasdale, J. D. (1997, July). *Preventing depressive relapse: Applying ICS to ACT*. Paper presented at the British Association for Behavioural and Cognitive Psychotherapies conference, Canterbury, UK.

Teasdale, J. D. (1999a). Emotional processing, three modes of mind and the prevention of relapse in depression. *Behaviour Research and Therapy, 37*, S53–S58.

Teasdale, J. D. (1999b). Multi-level theories of cognition-emotion relations. In T. Dalgleish & M. J. Power (Eds.), *Handbook of cognition and emotion* (pp. 665–682). Chichester, UK: Wiley.

Teasdale, J. D. (2004). Mindfulness-based cognitive therapy. In J. Yiend (Ed.), *Cognition, emotion and psychopathology* (pp. 270–289). Cambridge, UK: Cambridge University Press.

Teasdale, J. D., & Barnard, P. J. (1993). *Affect, cognition and change*. Hove, UK: Erlbaum.

Teasdale, J. D., Segal, Z. V., Williams, J. M. G., Ridgeway, V., Soulsby, J., & Lau, M. (2000). Reducing risk of recurrence of major depression using mindfulness-based cognitive therapy. *Journal of Consulting and Clinical Psychology, 68*, 615–623.

van der Kolk, B. A. (1994). The body keeps the score: Memory and the evolving psychobiology of posttraumatic stress. *Harvard Review of Psychiatry, 1*, 253–265.

Wade, C., & Tavris, C. (1993). *Psychology* (3rd ed.). New York: HarperCollins.

Warwick, H. M. C., & Salkovskis, P. M. (1990). Hypochondriasis. *Behaviour Research and Therapy, 28*, 105–117.

Warwick, H. M. C., & Salkovskis, P. M. (2001). Cognitive-behavioural treatment of hypochondriasis. In V. Starcevic & D. R. Lipsitt (Eds.), *Hypochondriasis: Modern perspectives on an ancient malady* (pp. 202–222). New York: Oxford University Press.

Watkins, J. G. (1971). *Hypnoanalytical techniques: The practice of clinical hypnosis* (Vol. II). New York: Irvington.

Weertman, A., & Arntz, A. (2007). Effectiveness of treatment of childhood memories in cognitive therapy for personality disorders: A controlled study contrasting methods focusing on the present and methods focusing on childhood memories. *Behaviour Research and Therapy, 45*, 2133–2143.

Wegner, D. A., Schneider, D., Carter, S. R., & White, T. L. (1987). Paradoxical effects of thought suppression. *Journal of Personality and Social Psychology, 53*, 5–13.

Weitzman, B. (1967). Behaviour therapy and psychotherapy. *Psychological Review, 74*, 300–317.

Wells, A. (1995). Meta-cognition and worry: A cognitive model of generalized anxiety disorder. *Behavioural and Cognitive Psychotherapy, 23*, 301–320.

Wells, A. (1997). *Cognitive therapy of anxiety disorders: A practical manual and conceptual guide*. Chichester, UK: Wiley.

Wells, A. (2000). *Emotional disorders and metacognition: Innovative cognitive therapy*. Chichester, UK: Wiley.

Wells, A. (2002). Worry, metacognition, and GAD: Nature, consequences and treatment. *Journal of Cognitive Psychotherapy, 16*, 179–192.

Wells, A., & Clark, D. M. (1997). Social phobia: A cognitive approach. In G. C. L. Davey (Ed.), *Phobias: A handbook of theory, research and treatment* (pp. 3–26). Chichester, UK: Wiley.

Wells, A., & Hackmann, A. (1993). Imagery and core beliefs in health anxiety: Content and origins. *Behavioural and Cognitive Psychotherapy, 21*, 265–273.

Wells, A., & Mathews, G. (1994). *Attention and emotion: A clinical perspective*. Hove, UK: Erlbaum.

Wells, A., & Mathews, G. (1996). Modeling cognition in emotional disorder: The S-REF model. *Behaviour Research and Therapy, 32*, 867–880.

Wells, A., & Papageorgiou, C. (1995). Worry and the incubation of intrusive images following stress. *Behaviour Research and Therapy, 33*, 579–583.

Westbrook, D., Kennerley, H., & Kirk, J. (2007). *An introduction to cognitive behaviour therapy*. London: Sage.

Westbrook, D., & Kirk, J. (2005). The clinical effectiveness of cognitive behaviour therapy: Outcome for a large sample of adults treated in routine practice. *Behaviour Research and Therapy, 43*, 1243–1261.

Wheatley, J., Brewin, C. R., Patel, T., & Hackmann, A. (2007). "I'll believe it when I can see it":

Imagery re-scripting of intrusive sensory memories in depression. *Journal of Behavior Therapy and Experimental Psychiatry, 38*, 371–385.

Wild, J., Hackmann, A., & Clark, D. M. (2007). Rescripting early memories linked to negative images in social phobia: A pilot study. *Journal of Behavior Therapy and Experimental Psychiatry, 38*, 386–401.

Williams, J. M. G., Watts, F. N., MacLeod, C., & Mathews, A. (1997). *Cognitive psychology and emotional disorders* (2nd ed.). Chichester, UK: Wiley.

Wolpe, J. (1958). *Psychotherapy by reciprocal inhibition*. Palo Alto, CA: Stanford University Press.

Yiend, J. (2004). *Cognition, emotion and psychopathology: Theoretical, empirical and clinical directions*. Cambridge, UK: Cambridge University Press.

Young, J. (1990). *Cognitive therapy for personality disorders: A schema-focused approach*. Sarasota, FL: Professional Resource Exchange.

Young, J. E., Klosko, J. S., & Weishaar, M. E. (2003). *Schema therapy: A practitioner's guide*. New York: Guilford Press.

Index

Page numbers followed by *f* indicate figure, *t* indicate table.

218